Miracle Babies

& Other Happy Endings
for Couples with
Fertility Problems

Miracle Babies

& Other Happy Endings
for Couples with
Fertility Problems

Mark Perloe, M.D.,
and Linda Gail Christie

RAWSON ASSOCIATES
New York

To Laura Perloe
and Jennifer and Stephen Christie
for helping us realize
the importance of miracle babies

Library of Congress Cataloging-in-Publication Data

Perloe, Mark.
  Miracle babies and other happy endings for
couples with fertility problems.

  Includes index.
  1. Infertility—Popular works. I. Christie, Linda
Gail. II. Title. [DNLM: 1. Infertility—therapy—popular
works. WP 570 P451m]
RC889.P37   1986   618.1'78   85-43088
ISBN 0-89256-301-X

Published simultaneously in Canada by Collier Macmillan Canada, Inc.
Packaged by Rapid Transcript, a division of March Tenth, Inc.
Composition by Folio Graphics
Printed and bound by Fairfield Graphics, Fairfield, Pennsylvania
Designed by Jacques Chazaud
Illustrations furnished by Serono Laboratories, Inc. and
drawn by Bill Lange.
First Edition

Contents

Acknowledgments

The authors wish to thank the many people who contributed their time and expertise to this book.

The members of the Tulsa chapter of RESOLVE, Inc., provided the inspiration and understanding we needed to communicate our message. They also generously shared their experiences with infertility—their concerns, their fears, and their joys. Throughout this book you will have an opportunity to benefit from the knowledge of these truly brave and remarkable people.

We also received expert technical advice and assistance from Steve Ackerman, Ph.D., Doris Baker, M.S., M.T. (ASCP), Gary Bullard, Ben Faulkner, J.D., Nancy G. Feldman, J.D., P. M. Fielding, Susan Leichtman, Donald R. Tredway, M.D., and Carol Walters, R.N.C. Dr. Perloe's patients and staff were very supportive and contributed much to the quality of this work.

We appreciate the generosity of Serono Laboratories, which funded the illustrations for this book. Our artist, Bill Lange, did a superb job. We also appreciate the support we received from the University of Oklahoma Tulsa Medical College.

We thank Robin Rue, our literary agent, who had enough faith in this project to hold out for an excellent publisher and editor. Our deepest appreciation goes to our editors, Eleanor Rawson and Toni Sciarra, who pushed our writing abilities to the limit and then asked for more.

We also wish to thank our families, especially our spouses, John Christie and Mary Perloe, who had to manage without us during the many hours needed to complete this project.

What This Book
Will Reveal to You

At this moment an epidemic is sweeping the country. Your friends won't be calling you to find out if you've fallen victim. Charitable organizations won't be formed to rush to your aid.

No. If you're having fertility problems, you probably feel that you're completely alone in your struggle. Your reaction may be, "Why me? Everyone else is having babies. It's not fair."

In my ten years of medical practice I have seen many infertile couples experience repeated disappointment, frustration, and disorientation. They cycle between guilt, anger, and despair—trapped in hope that with each new round of treatment they will conceive. When a course of therapy fails to produce a pregnancy, they experience all the stages of mourning—as though they had actually lost an infant.

Over the years, however, I have seen many couples learn to deal with their trauma. They manage to get control of their lives and their feelings. They take an active part in their diagnosis and treatment. In fact, they seem to grow stronger and closer as a result of struggling with their fertility problem. It is because of these people that I decided to write this book.

I want to tell you not only how these couples coped but also how they resolved their fertility problems. I hope that by sharing their experiences, you will gain insight into your parenting needs and be able to design a course of treatment and therapy that will meet those goals. In addition, you will avoid unnecessary procedures, unwarranted disappointments, and excessive costs. Above all, you will feel less like a victim and, I hope, much less alone.

I want to assure you that your fertility problems, your anger, your hypersensitivity, your feelings of inadequacy, and your eternal optimism aren't unique to *just you*. Fertility problems strike one in six American couples—4.5 million people. Each year over 1 million people consult physicians for infertility evaluation and treatment.

The medical definition of infertility is "the inability to conceive after a year of unprotected intercourse or the inability to carry a pregnancy to term." However, if you already know or suspect that you have a fertility problem, you should seek an evaluation before waiting a year while trying to conceive. For example, a woman may suspect a problem if she suffers extreme pain with menstruation, has a history of pelvic inflammatory disease, or has few menstrual periods. A man may be concerned if he has ever contracted a sexually transmitted disease, has symptoms of genitourinary tract infection, or has an undescended or injured testicle. *Infertility should not be confused with sterility,* which is an irreversible condition. And it should not be referred to as *subfertility,* which connotes a borderline fertility problem that may not require treatment. *All* fertility problems, however, should be evaluated to determine their seriousness.

Recently I have witnessed astounding progress in the diagnosis and treatment of infertility. Only a few years ago most couples with fertility problems had to turn to adoption or remain childless. But now, with the advances in pharmaceuticals, microsurgery, in vitro fertilization, and embryo transfer, many viable options have opened up to infertile couples—with the result that "miracle babies" are being born almost every day. *There is every reason for hope.*

I hope to help satisfy your thirst for medically sound information about your infertility—what may have caused it, what tests are available to diagnose the causes, what can be done to correct the problems, and most important, what your options are. Being informed of the most up-to-date medical technology will help you work with your physician to develop an effective, individualized course of treatment.

It is not uncommon to find fertility problems in both partners. However, even when only one of you must be medically treated, I find that the fertility problem affects both of you because the *couple* loses control of their destiny, the *couple* undergoes fertility treatment, and the *couple* shares the emotional strain of dealing with friends and family. Infertility does not affect just one person—*it affects the couple.*

Most people respond to infertility with disbelief and anger. As infertility becomes a reality, as they begin medical treatment, and if they experience repeated failures, their anxiety and frustration grow. *All* infertile couples suffer psychological trauma. *All* infertile couples feel cheated. *All* infertile couples feel that they've lost control of one of their most personal rights—the right to bear children. If you suffer from these symptoms, *you are not alone.*

In this book I will help you rethink the myths that may be haunting you and interfering with your self-esteem, your sexuality, and your progress toward conception. I want to help you stabilize your life so that you can deal with other important, related aspects of your life—your marriage, your family, your friends, and your career. You are entitled to have the freedom to be yourself and to consider new options apart from what others expect or demand. You may even want to give your family and friends a copy of this book so they can become more sensitive to your needs.

I will also inform you of the legal controversies surrounding the latest technologies for infertility treatment. You will learn why attorneys and lawmakers are concerned and even confused about parenting rights, fetal rights, and custody definitions when it comes to miracle baby making. With this information you will be able to sort through the moral and ethical decisions you may face regarding issues such as artificial insemination, in vitro fertilization, and genetic counseling.

I believe that by reading this book, you will find encouragement, understanding, comfort, practical solutions, and the courage to keep trying for your own miracle baby.

> Mark Perloe, M.D.
> Fellow of the American College of
>   Obstetricians and Gynecologists
> Diplomate of the American Board of
>   Obstetrics and Gynecology
> Member, American Fertility Society
>
> Columbia, Maryland

Miracle Babies

& Other Happy Endings
for Couples with
Fertility Problems

1. How I Discovered the Secrets of Successful Fertility Treatment

I began to grow skeptical about the accepted methods for infertility treatment when I realized that I wasn't meeting the needs of my patients. Although I was investing a lot of energy and emotion into their problems, I was becoming more and more frustrated with the way they responded to my care.

Many of my patients acted as if they didn't hear my instructions. For example, every time I told Lori I'd have her test results in three days, she'd call me the next morning for the results. When I tried to schedule an ultrasound examination for Debbie, she'd either cancel at the last minute or simply not show up. Bridgette wasn't able to maintain a basal temperature chart and Jennifer always forgot to bring her temperature chart to her appointment. I couldn't understand why these intelligent and highly motivated people acted so erratically.

The reasons became clear once I discovered how my patients blossomed when they became *a positive force in their infertility treatment*. I'd like to share with you how I uncovered these secrets and how you can benefit from my formula for success.

"I feel like a guinea pig."

Growing frustration forced me to rethink my approach with infertile couples. One day Cheryl said, "I feel like a guinea pig. This whole business is dehumanizing." She broke down and cried, and I wasn't sure what I could do for her. Moreover, I was completely surprised when her husband not only refused to cooperate but even *blamed* me for her inability to get pregnant!

In retrospect, I realize that I not only underestimated the stress my patients were experiencing but I may have even contributed to their frustration. In my clumsy attempts to defuse their depression with humor, I remember saying such insensitive things as, "You can borrow my kid for the weekend," or, "At least you don't have trouble finding baby-sitters."

I wasn't the only one who didn't know what to say to infertile couples. Their families, friends, and co-workers always seemed to be in error, too; even a concerned inquiry about their infertility treatment stirred anger and anxiety. I observed that as treatments extended into months and sometimes into years, my patients seemed to become less communicative and more paranoid. Some even went so far as to isolate themselves from others.

In my quest for answers to these problems I instinctively turned to the literature for guidance. When I checked the local bookstores, I found that infertility books offered few concrete suggestions. Popular literature tended to be cold, technical reproductive biology texts or too generalized to be useful.

My search continued until I saw a newspaper advertisement for an infertility seminar conducted by RESOLVE, Inc., and Serono Laboratories. RE-SOLVE is a nationwide, nonprofit support organization for infertile couples. What I learned from RESOLVE and subsequent studies changed my whole approach to infertility practice.

I became aware that in the face of a diagnosis of infertility many people experience as much or more trauma than people who are told that they suffer from a life-threatening disease. Typical are Bret and Nancy L., who discovered they were infertile in their early thirties. Feeling trapped by circumstance, they became angry and depressed. They felt guilty about their use of birth control pills for ten years. The ten-year "delay" shortened the number of fertile years Nancy had for treatment, and her increased age reduced her chances for pregnancy even further. They had always had some problems communicating with each other, and their complex and demanding treatment regimen began to aggravate the strain. My requests for temperature charts, semen analyses, and scheduled intercourse only seemed to add to their frustrations.

I realized that in order to establish a positive physician-patient relationship, I also had to address the emotional needs of patients like Bret and Nancy. Since I knew that much of their stress resulted from perceived loss of control, I developed a method that *put them back in control of every stage of their infertility treatment*. It was a method that improved their communications, provided feedback to my staff and me, and provided better treatment. Most of all, it was a method that improved their sense of self-worth.

My Five-Point Strategy for Fertility Treatment

Because *victims make poor patients,* I selected *restoration of control* as the starting point of my plan. To put my patients in charge of their infertility, I instituted the following procedures.

1. *I try to involve both partners in the initial discussions and planning.* In these meetings we discuss their medical histories and family goals. We talk

about diagnostic alternatives, medical resources, realistic timing, and emotional, time, and financial commitments. I answer their questions and give them the medical information that will help them think through their motives and alternatives. I want both of them to begin fertility treatment with realistic expectations and mutual understanding. I have found that this *planning phase* is so critical to successful fertility treatment that I've devoted several chapters of this book to showing how you can implement this process on your own. A jointly designed plan puts my patients back in control of their treatment, their bodies, and their immediate future. They no longer complain of being victims or guinea pigs. And they view me as a skilled partner or facilitator who is enhancing their effort to achieve pregnancy.

2. *I offer recommendations instead of mandates.* As their partner, I suggest diagnostic procedures and courses of treatment for consideration. I discuss alternatives, side effects, the odds for success, and other relevant issues. My patients *choose* their course of action.

3. *I tailor my testing and treatment to their emotional needs and budgets.* Some patients want to proceed at breakneck speed, while others are more comfortable with a relaxed approach. I try to adjust my scheduling to their comfort level, and I always consult with them before altering our agreed-upon strategy. A number of patients find that they must adjust their treatment to accommodate their financial resources. An overextended budget only adds to their anxiety and usually isn't necessary for effective treatment. I also help them explore what expenses may be covered by insurance.

4. *I make certain that either my nurse practitioner or I am always accessible to answer questions and offer support.* Together we can provide the time, information, and consulting skills that our patients need.

5. *I refer most of my patients to the local RESOLVE chapter for information, peer support, and, if desired, group counseling.* I'm very impressed with the quality of information, printed material, and support offered by RESOLVE. The most important service it offers is understanding, companionship, and acceptance. Only in this kind of environment can infertile couples feel that they are not alone in the world and that their feelings are normal. And they can learn effective coping skills from others who are experiencing similar problems. You will learn many of these skills throughout this book.

I know that this five-point approach will work for you because my patients have done so well. Once they see the difference the plan makes in their lives, they seldom experience the trauma I had so frequently observed when I dealt with infertile couples. I remember one patient saying, "I didn't know that I could deal with infertility treatment as just another one of life's hurdles. Our problems used to seem so monumental before Don and I put our goals and treatment plan on paper."

The next few chapters will show you step by step how to lay the groundwork for such a successful plan. Successive chapters will help you:

- Become informed about the most up-to-date medical information so you will know how to choose the right physician and how to tell if you are getting the best treatment
- Develop an individualized treatment plan with your physician so you can take an active part in your diagnosis and medical care
- Get control of your life and feelings of anxiety so you can stop making impossible demands on yourself and others
- Become a positive force in your fertility treatment
- Identify your "happy ending" and pursue it

So now let's begin to identify the ingredients for *your* happy ending.

I. Making Your Fertility Treatment Plan

2. Taking Control of Your Fertility

Take a moment to think about your married life before you thought you had a fertility problem. You were happy, optimistic, and looking forward to the day when together you'd create a new life—when you would begin your family. For one reason or another you may have delayed starting one. You may have saved for a house, finished college, taken your dream vacation, or begun a career. You wanted the best possible start for your marriage before you settled down to enjoy having a family.

Then the roof caved in.

"I remember being surrounded by X rays. My mind wandered back to the day Mitch and I decided to wait to have a baby. I had wanted to start my public relations career. We had been able to buy our dream house where our babies could play in their own backyard. As the doctor pointed to the shadowy pictures, he explained how my blocked tubes were preventing my pregnancy. I don't remember much more after that—only my pain and disappointment."

Jeanne is only one of my patients who, late in her reproductive life, discovered a fertility problem. Fortunately, soon after I repaired her damaged fallopian tubes with microsurgery, Jeanne and Mitch conceived and had a beautiful, normal baby boy. She's now pregnant with her second baby.

In my practice I have found that many couples' problems aren't resolved as quickly as Jeanne's. Their diagnosis may be more elusive, their treatment more complex. For example, by the time Michael and Shelley T. came to me, they both were discouraged and worried. For two years they had been trying unsuccessfully to conceive. Their physician had already completed a fertility workup, performed painful tubal surgery, and prescribed powerful fertility drugs—all to no avail. When I first saw them, their quality of life had deteriorated to an unfortunate low.

5

The advice that I gave Michael and Shelley worked for them and *it will work for you, too.* I'm going to show you how you can permanently improve your quality of life, even when faced with overwhelming odds. And I'm certain that as a couple you will grow closer and stronger from your efforts.

Couples You Will Meet in This Book

In this book you will become acquainted with four couples who took charge of their fertility problems and found their miracle babies:

Michael and Shelley T.

When her doctor recommended a hysterectomy, Shelley T. panicked. She was afraid that Michael would divorce her because she thought that having a baby was the most important thing a wife could do for him.

By the time I saw them, all Michael could do was grumble about mounting medical bills; he thought all fertility specialists were "rip-off artists." Shelley was hurt, angry, and distrustful. She'd put her life and her career on hold, believing that "I'd get pregnant any day." The only reason she had requested a second opinion was the encouragement she received from the RESOLVE infertility support group when they heard that Michael had never had a semen analysis.

By blindly accepting one test and treatment after another, this couple had forfeited their responsibility and control for their fertility. Michael's lack of interest and support not only added to Shelley's difficulties but, as it turned out, also prevented an accurate diagnosis—he had no sperm in his semen. She had undergone years of expensive treatment, but never had a chance for pregnancy. Their situation illustrates what can happen when you have unrealistic expectations and pursue no clear-cut treatment plan.

In this book you will see how Shelley and Michael took control of their fertility treatment and their lives. And you will find out how they got their miracle baby, Tommy.

Bryan and Debbie W.

Debbie believed that until she had a baby she would not be a complete woman. When spontaneous bleeding disrupted her third month of pregnancy, Debbie became desperate: "I've already lost two babies. If I lose another, I don't know what I'll do." Unfortunately after her spontaneous abortion began, there wasn't much I could do to save their baby. But I could do a lot to keep her from losing their next baby.

In later chapters you will learn how Debbie and Bryan coped with their loss and grief. And you'll learn how Debbie's exposure to DES, while she was still in her mother's womb, destined her for repeated abortions.

When I secured Debbie's incompetent cervix during her next pregnancy, she was able to have a beautiful blue-eyed baby girl.

Steven and Kathy S.

Kathy's periods probably stopped because of the excess running she did to prepare for amateur competition. Running, however, was very important to Kathy's self-image. She wanted to maintain her life-style and have a baby, too.

"Before we commit to a bunch of tests, we want to know what to expect," Kathy S. said on their first visit. "We want a baby, but we have our lives to live, too." Kathy and Steven wanted to understand the big picture: what tests I'd recommend, what the results would mean, how long it would take, what the odds were that she'd conceive, and what it would cost.

After the initial workup, they were surprised to find that Steven had a poor semen analysis. I suspected that his varicocoele (varicose vein in the scrotum) might also be impairing their ability to have a child.

As their story unfolds, you will find out how this couple's take-control attitude and their desire for having a fertility treatment plan led them on a direct path toward their goal.

You will also find out how their persistence and hard work during ovulation induction treatment eventually paid off.

Richard and Margaret B.

Since graduating from college, Margaret had pursued a successful career. When she was thirty-one she and Richard decided that she should stop taking the Pill so they could begin their family. But nothing happened.

Concerned about their progress, a year later Margaret came to me requesting a fertility evaluation. Although her physical examination revealed no obvious fertility problem, I was concerned about possible complications from the ruptured appendix she had suffered at twenty-three. The tubal X ray confirmed my suspicions: it revealed that both of Margaret's tubes were blocked.

When I received the results of Richard's semen analysis, I became concerned that his consistent use of marijuana could be impairing his fertility potential.

In this book you will find out how even though microsurgery restored Margaret's fallopian tubes, the surgery did not make her fertile. And you will learn how the miracle of in vitro fertilization gave them the son they wanted so much.

Seeing how each of these couples managed their fertility problems will provide you with insight into the many options you have in coping with infertility and its treatment.

The steps I recommend for planning a fertility treatment program make common sense and are easy to follow. As you learn more about your fertility and about your treatment, you will become less tense and anxious. You will be able to formulate a short-term plan and set long-term goals as well.

Together with your physician, you will be able to take an active part in your individualized diagnosis and treatment.

Dispelling the Eleven Worst Myths About Infertility

The first step involves rethinking a lot of the myths you have been taught about fertility problems.

Myth #1: Infertility Is the Woman's Problem

For years physicians and infertile couples believed that fertility problems stemmed primarily from the woman. In fact, suspected barrenness was a man's grounds for divorce as well as a king's justification for beheading his wife. Today, however, we know that fertility problems are *equally common* in both men and women. Although the statistics vary some from study to study, the consensus is that it's the woman's problem about one-third of the time and the man's problem about one-third of the time. In 5 to 10 percent of the cases, the causes can't be clearly identified. The balance of the cases stem from deficiencies in *both* partners. This was most dramatically illustrated by Kathy, who had ovulatory problems, while her husband, Steven, had a varicocoele that interfered with his sperm production.

We now know that performing surgery on a woman married to a man with a dramatically low sperm count won't improve the odds for pregnancy. You can achieve pregnancy only when *both* partners are contributing the proper ingredients at the proper time. In the following chapters you will learn more about how this miracle occurs.

Myth #2: Infertility Can Be Cured by Taking a Vacation

Although stress and tension may interfere with your sexual desires and with your performance in the bedroom, there's no scientific evidence that your emotional state directly causes your fertility problem. While menstrual irregularities may be the result of stress and tension, these irregularities can be medically corrected, so that stress need not affect your fertility.

Conversely, there's no reason why your fertility problem should affect your performance in the bedroom. I remember Steve and Kathy saying; "Sex for pleasure? What's that?" Later in this book you will discover how they managed to restore pleasure to sex and how you can, too.

Myth #3: If You're Fertile, You Should Get Pregnant in Two Months

In a normal population of couples who are trying to conceive, each couple will have a 20 percent chance of getting pregnant the first month. Odds are funny: the remaining 80 percent who didn't conceive the first month have the same chances the next month—only 20 percent of that 80 percent will get pregnant.

For example, if one hundred couples try to get pregnant in January, approximately twenty will conceive. That leaves eighty to try again in February. In February 20 percent, or sixteen, of them will be successful, leaving sixty-six who will have to try in March. In March 20 percent of those will become pregnant (approximately fourteen), leaving fifty-two for April. So, in three months, roughly half of our hundred couples have conceived, *but another half have not conceived.* At this rate, after seven months twenty-two people still will not have conceived, and after two years 10 to 15 percent still will not have conceived.

Unless they have reason to suspect there's a problem, I recommend to my patients that they not be overly concerned about their fertility until they have been unsuccessful for a full year. In fact, it sometimes happens that a couple conceives during the fertility workup without my otherwise doing anything— I'm a benefactor of the odds, you might say. I enjoy this kind of surprise.

The odds for conceiving are especially disconcerting to fertility patients whose problems have been corrected. For example, Steven and Kathy thought that their first artificial insemination treatment (using Steven's sperm) would do the trick. I had to caution them that it might take as many as ten or twelve cycles for them to achieve a pregnancy.

When I reflect on how complicated human reproduction is, I sometimes wonder how most women get pregnant. Nature did not design the human reproductive system so that a woman could get pregnant at the drop of a hat. Later in this book you will find out why our reproductive systems are so inefficient. You will also learn about the most up-to-date diagnostic procedures and corrective treatments available, including in vitro fertilization, frozen embryo transplants, and surrogate wombs. You have many options for improving your odds for conception.

Myth #4: If You Adopt, You'll Get Pregnant

Statistics show that 5 to 10 percent of adoptive couples conceive. I firmly believe, however, that these people would have conceived anyway, regardless of the adoption. As we already know, many couples with fertility problems eventually conceive without any medical intervention. Richard and Margaret almost opted for adoption until I convinced them that they were responding to an old wives' tale, because their secret hope was that adoption would "cause" a pregnancy.

Some adoptive couples choose to continue with their fertility treatment. Their adoptive child satisfies their parenting needs, but doesn't satisfy the couple's desire to produce a genetic heir. These couples may also eventually achieve a pregnancy.

Myth #5: Once You're Infertile, You're Always Infertile

I have observed that when many couples receive the diagnosis of infertility, they just give up. They don't think that the tests, drugs, surgery, and all of their effort will be worth it.

About 5 to 10 percent of these people will conceive without medical intervention. However, *50 percent or more* could benefit from fertility treatment. *Making* a miracle instead of *waiting* for a miracle is the answer if you really want a child.

Myth #6: Fertility Is a Sign of Virility

Many men feel that fertility problems threaten their manliness. In fact, some husbands go so far as to refuse a simple semen analysis, as Michael T. had in the past. He was concerned about finding out that he "wasn't a man." Once he learned why the test was so important for diagnosing their fertility problem, he agreed to take it.

Since in approximately two-thirds of my cases the man's fertility may be the cause, I insist that the male have a semen analysis.

Fertility and sexual function are not necessarily related. In cases where severe hormone deficiencies, physical damage, physical deformity, medical illness, or drug usage exist, sexual dysfunction may be the reason why pregnancy hasn't occurred. However, I find that this is relatively rare.

Myth #7: You Caused Your Miscarriage

We know that 10 to 15 percent of confirmed pregnancies will miscarry. When we examine the fetus, we find that 60 percent have one-time-event genetic abnormalities. Sometimes a placenta develops, but no fetus is present. This will produce a positive pregnancy test but obviously will not produce a baby. Miscarriage is nature's way of discarding a deformed embryo or fetus so a viable pregnancy can begin. The likelihood that a miscarriage will occur with the next pregnancy is once again 10 to 15 percent.

I find that repeated pregnancy loss may indicate a pathological problem such as an incompetent cervix or adhesions (scars) inside the uterus. Later chapters will tell you how I successfully treated Debbie W.'s problem with repeated pregnancy loss.

Myth #8: Long-term Contraceptive Use Causes Infertility

Many of you may be concerned that long-term use of oral contraceptives (birth control pills) or intrauterine devices (IUDs) may have impaired your fertility. I would like to address both of these issues.

Since the risks of infection and intrauterine scarring are increased with the use of an IUD, I no longer insert IUDs, and I recommend their removal, particularly for women who wish to have children.

When IUD use results in infertility, as it did in Richard and Margaret B.'s case, we have a number of options for repairing the damage. You will learn how Richard and Margaret's treatment resulted in the birth of a healthy baby boy.

With respect to using oral contraceptives, I advise my patients who have menstrual irregularity prior to using oral contraceptives that they may have an underlying fertility problem. This problem will probably grow no worse, but neither will it improve with the use of oral contraceptives. Studies have shown that after the cessation of birth control pills, up to 3 percent of women will experience ovulatory problems. These women usually respond very well to treatment. Problems conceiving that are often attributed to long-term use of the Pill are, in my opinion, more likely due to the fact that as women grow older, their odds for getting pregnant deteriorate naturally. Because Margaret and Richard waited until their mid-thirties to start their family, they had to face this problem.

Some experts feel that the normal aging of the reproductive organs diminishes fertility. Others feel that the longer you wait to conceive, the more you risk reducing fertility through infections, use of IUDs, or surgeries. In addition, with age you have an increased risk of developing endometriosis (a condition in which for unknown reasons pieces of uterine lining adhere to pelvic organs and "bleed" with each monthly cycle). In later chapters you will learn more about how each of these factors can affect your fertility. Table 2-1 shows what your odds are for pregnancy at various ages, assuming that you have no serious fertility problems.

As you can see, regardless of the causes, fertility decreases with age. If you know that you may have a problem (for example, if your periods are irregular or you experience extreme pain during your periods), you shouldn't delay having a fertility evaluation.

Myth #9: Therapeutic Abortions Frequently Cause Infertility

Over 1 million abortions are performed in the United States each year. When abortions were illegal, performed by amateurs, and conducted in septic conditions, sterility and even death were common. However, with sterile conditions and professional medical supervision, the first-trimester abortion presents minimal risk for decreased fertility. Repeated abortions, however, may increase your likelihood for early pregnancy loss, premature birth, and failure to conceive.

Table 2-1
The Relationship Between Age and Fertility

Odds of Getting Pregnant Each Month and During the First Year

Age	% Pregnancy Per Month	% Pregnancy First Year
Early 20s	20–25	94
Late 20s and early 30s	10–15	70–85
Late 30s	8–10	65–70

Odds of Getting Pregnant During the First Six Months

Age	% Pregnancy
25	75
Late 20s	47
Early 30s	38
Late 30s	25
40	22

Average Time to Conception

Age	Months
Early 20s	4–5
Late 20s	5–7
Early 30s	7–10
Late 30s	10–12

Myth #10: A Free-Style Sex Life Leads to Infertility

You may have been told that your "escapades" before getting married led to your undoing. This is not necessarily true. There is no evidence that having sex with multiple partners or having sex prior to marriage causes infertility. In fact, you may be surprised to know that as long ago as 1979, over two-thirds of never-married women had had sexual intercourse by the time they were nineteen years old.

However, having sex with multiple partners *does* increase your risk of contracting sexually transmitted infections (gonorrhea, chlamydia, urea-plasma, condyloma, etc.), which may cause pelvic inflammatory disease (PID). One million women will contract PID this year and a quarter of them will require hospitalization due to the severity of the disease. If you contract PID *once,* you have up to a 20 percent chance of developing a fertility problem. This means that 150,000 to 200,000 women exposed to chlamydia or gonorrhea will become infertile this year.

What makes these diseases so insidious is that you may not have any overt symptoms. So until you fail to get pregnant, you may not even know that your tubes have been severely scarred from infection.

I recommend to my patients that they request a pelvic exam if they have any pain, midcycle bleeding, or other abnormal symptoms. Otherwise, as the American College of Obstetricians and Gynecologists recommends, I suggest that my patients have an annual pelvic exam which screens not only for cancer but also for gonorrhea.

Myth #11: A Rise in Your Basal Temperature Means You're Fertile

Many of my patients report that they have been scheduling sexual intercourse to correspond to their rise in basal body temperature, as Margaret and Richard did. Having intercourse *after* Margaret's temperature rose, however, almost guaranteed that she would *not* get pregnant. In effect, they were practicing good rhythm birth control. They were having intercourse twenty-four hours too late!

You are fertile for about twenty-four hours during each ovulatory cycle. A rise in your basal temperature signifies that your ovary is secreting progesterone—an event that occurs twenty-four hours *after* ovulation. For conception to take place, the sperm must be present immediately before or at the time of ovulation.

I ask my patients to keep a temperature chart to help me verify that they actually are ovulating with each cycle. Later, you will find out more about how you can predict when you are fertile and how we can detect what's really happening with your hormones, ovaries, and eggs. In addition, you'll learn how we can control these factors to optimize your chances for conception.

An Infertility Management Plan Will Help Stabilize Your Life

Your own physician is your best ally in the battle against infertility. To take full advantage of his or her skills, however, you *must* take an active part in your therapy: inform your physician of your symptoms, ask questions, make suggestions, and explore alternatives. Having done this, it becomes much easier to understand and better accept his or her recommendations. Help your physician understand what you're experiencing.

"I should be happy, but I'm not."

Your plan should address not only your fertility problems; it should also attend to your psychological needs—your depression, your anger, your frustration, your feelings of inadequacy. These feelings are absolutely *normal*. In fact, I'd think something was wrong with you if you *didn't* have them.

I'll show you how other couples have overcome their disappointments and have learned to go on with their lives.

Your plan should also help you deal with your well-meaning but often insensitive relatives, friends, and co-workers. How many times have you heard, "You should be happy. Look at how fortunate you are. You've got everything *else* anyone could want." Their attempts to comfort you only heighten your anger and widen the communication gap. I'll share with you how other couples have dealt with these people and how they've learned to live in a world full of babies and pregnant women.

Think about your married life before you knew you were infertile. If you want to return to that happy, optimistic life, keep reading!

3. Finding
Your Happy Ending

"Without children life would be meaningless."

"I don't have anything in common with my friends who have children. Being different makes me uncomfortable."

"A baby will make our marriage happier and more stable."

"Fitting meetings, graduate school, and business trips into feedings, diapers, and baby-sitters would stifle me."

"Pregnant women glow with their femininity."

I have heard all of these statements and more from patients and friends—normal men and women with normal feelings and concerns. I find, however, that many of my fertility patients are afraid to explore or discuss their feelings—both positive and negative—about having children. They are so intent on resolving their fertility problems—on *creating a pregnancy*—that they lose sight that what they are really trying to do is *make a baby*. They seldom stop to ask themselves, "Why?" and, "How is this baby going to change our relationship and lives?" and, "Do I welcome those changes—*or most of them*—wholeheartedly?"

A fertility treatment plan should lead to results that will satisfy your basic needs. Since the happy ending that's right for you may be different from the one that another may choose, *it is vital at the outset that you both identify how having a baby will meet your needs*. Will the baby carry on your family name and genes? Will having the baby make you feel like a complete person? Will the baby be your companion—someone to nurture and love?

The answers to these and other questions will greatly influence your treatment options. If like Steven and Kathy you want a baby to carry on the family name and genes, donor artificial insemination will not be a happy ending for you. If like Debbie you want to carry a pregnancy to make your life experience complete, then adoption won't be a happy ending. But if you just want a baby to nurture and love, as Richard and Margaret did, you won't be as concerned with *how* you get your baby as with just getting one.

Evaluating Your Desire
to Have a Baby

To help you identify your happy ending, I have developed an evaluation test for you and your spouse. I use it with my patients before we sit down to work out a fertility plan. Discussing your responses with one another will help you understand your motives, concerns, interests, attitudes, and feelings. You will both gain insight into why your fertility problems cause you pain and frustration. And you will be able to identify which happy ending will resolve your fertility problem.

Even my patients who have been receiving fertility treatment for a year or more enjoy and benefit from taking this test. "When we discussed our answers to the test, it was the first time we'd talked about our problem when we weren't in the middle of a crisis," Shelley T. reported. "It was very refreshing."

I recommend that my patients retake the evaluation every six months or so. This renews their dialogue and identifies significant changes in their attitudes. People like Michael and Shelley who at first completely rule out adoption, for example, will often find that it becomes more attractive after years of unsuccessful treatment.

It's okay to change your mind. If you don't achieve your first goal, you may wish to reexamine your needs and select another. You probably didn't succeed at getting a date with your first love either, but that didn't stop you from trying again or finding an alternative. Besides, you may not have had all of the facts when you made your initial decisions.

Once you have discussed your answers together, you will be better prepared to find medical and professional services that will meet your needs.

Since you may wish to use the evaluation test several times throughout your fertility treatment, I suggest that you write your answers on a separate piece of paper. Number the sheet from 1 to 70 for your responses. By placing your completed answer sheet beside your spouse's, you can easily identify points of agreement and conflict. You may wish to save your answers and discuss them from time to time and compare them with future scores.

When you respond to the statements, do not ponder too long on any one issue. I find that an initial response is often more accurate than one analyzed to death. You should be able to complete the test in just a few minutes. After that, I will tell you how to interpret your answers and what they mean to you, to your spouse, and to your fertility treatment.

Examining each of these areas will help you understand how internal and external forces influence your reaction to infertility. By tuning in to these forces you can learn to accept your emotional responses, choose to accept or ignore the needs of others, discover your spouse's needs, and together control your future.

An Evaluation:
Why Is It So Important for You to Have a Baby?

INSTRUCTIONS: Number a sheet of paper from 1 to 70. Beside each number rate how important each statement is to you. Zero (0) means that the statement is *not very important* or is *least descriptive* of you. Five (5) means that the statement is *very important* or *very descriptive* of you. Use the numbers between 0 and 5 to show gradations between these extremes. If the statement doesn't seem to apply to your situation, place an X beside it. *There are no right or wrong answers.* Have your spouse take the evaluation separately. Then compare the two answer sheets and discuss where you agree and differ.

1. Children bring couples closer together.
2. Couples without children eventually become less stable and dissatisfied.
3. I want to see my spouse enjoying children.
4. I want a baby because it's important to my spouse.
5. I'm afraid our infertility may threaten our marriage.
6. My spouse wants a child.
7. Infertility makes me feel inadequate.
8. Sometimes I fear pregnancy.
9. Having a baby will demonstrate my virility/femininity.
10. I want a baby so my genes will be immortal.
11. I may someday regret not having done everything possible to have a baby.
12. I want to create a new life in my image.
13. Infertility makes me feel cheated.
14. I want my child to achieve some of the things I haven't been able to.
15. I want children so they can give me love and affection.
16. Without children I feel lonely.
17. Without children I'm bored.
18. Without children life is meaningless.
19. My infertility makes me feel powerless.
20. Sometimes I feel that I'm too self-centered.
21. I want a baby so I can quit my job.
22. I want children because then there will never be a dull moment in my life.
23. I sometimes wonder if we can afford a baby.
24. Having a family is what life is all about.
25. I want a baby because we live so far away from family and old friends.
26. I want a child who can help with my business/housework/hobby.
27. I feel that a woman's role should be mother and homemaker.
28. I feel that a man's role should be father and breadwinner.
29. I feel we are economically secure.

30. I've looked forward to having children all my life.
31. We frequently run out of money between paychecks.
32. Both of us have full-time jobs we enjoy.
33. Children will interfere with my career.
34. Children will interfere with my freedom to travel, be spontaneous, and live in the style I'm accustomed to.
35. I'm not sure I want the responsibility of a child for the next twenty years.
36. There's never a "right" time for having a baby.
37. I'm not sure what to do with my life if I don't have a baby.
38. A child will not substantially affect our life-style.
39. I want a baby so I can show my spouse/father/mother/siblings that I can be a good parent.
40. I want a baby so my child will have a sibling.
41. I feel I'm breaking tradition by not having children.
42. People who can afford children should have children.
43. Infertility keeps me from fulfilling my religious beliefs.
44. I live in a community where everyone has children, a home, and a backyard.
45. I live in a city crowded with high-rise apartments.
46. I'll never really be perceived as an adult until I have children.
47. The family will treat us better when we give them grandchildren.
48. Having children will bring me respect and prestige.
49. I don't want the family name to end with me.
50. I can't face telling my family/friends about our infertility.
51. Having and wanting children is natural.
52. Not having and not wanting children is unnatural.
53. Women have a maternal instinct that needs to be filled.
54. Denying maternal instinct denies a woman's basic nature and function.
55. Sacrificing for children is noble and unselfish.
56. Deciding to remain childless is selfish and immature.
57. Having children is a stage necessary for adult development.
58. Good parents have a lot of children.
59. People with a lot of money have more children.
60. People who don't want children don't have anything to offer them.
61. Infertility is God's/nature's way of limiting the population.
62. My (our) parents want us to have children.
63. I like to take care of children—feed, diaper, bathe, clothe, etc.
64. I like to play with children.
65. I want children so I can give them love and affection.
66. I want a baby because I think I will make a good parent.
67. I sometimes wonder if I will make a good parent.
68. Children are stimulating, novel, and fun.
69. I look forward to sharing my knowledge and experience with children.
70. I like to direct and control children.

What Your Answers Mean

The test is divided into five categories:

Statements	Subject
1–6	Couple needs or considerations
7–20	Internal needs (ego needs)
21–38	Life-style needs
39–62	External pressures (needs of others)
63–70	Parenting/nurturing needs

Couple Needs or Considerations
(Statements 1–6)

I find that most couples with fertility problems care for each other very much—perhaps too much. For example, Bryan W. said in a private interview, "I really don't care that much about having a baby. But I want one for Debbie's sake." When I interviewed Debbie, she said, "I'm afraid Bryan will divorce me and find a woman who can bear his children." In this case each misinterpreted the other's desires and was more concerned about the other's needs than his or her own. Their lack of communication and understanding added to their stress and hampered their choice of a mutually satisfying treatment program. When Bryan and Debbie began to share their feelings, they became happier and even more committed to finding a happy ending that was right for them. Comparing your test responses to your spouse's will help you see what is important to each of you instead of trying to outguess one another, as this couple had been doing.

The first six statements are designed to help you discover if you want a baby because *you think* your spouse wants one and/or because *you think* the success of your marriage depends upon having a baby. Believing that your marriage cannot survive without children is not unusual for an infertile couple. Shelley was so scared that she told me, "I will do *anything* to get pregnant—*no questions asked.*" Shelley answered "5" to all six of these questions. She was absolutely shocked, however, when Michael's answers indicated he wanted a baby *for her,* but that he did not feel their childlessness threatened their marriage. Shelley told me later, "This information helped us face and resolve some very basic communication problems."

Marriages actually do survive without children. In fact, population statistics indicate that marriages sometimes become *less* stable when children are introduced. The highest incidence of divorce occurs soon after the birth of the first child. I don't state this to frighten you, but to offer you some perspective. Children may *add* stress to a relationship because of their demands and impact on the couple's life-style. Moreover, the birth of a child will not stabilize an already rocky relationship.

As with Michael and Shelley, the foundation of your marriage may be stronger than you think. Knowing this will help you cope with your treatment and with your fertility in less emotional and distressing terms. If you both can focus your energy on developing and implementing a fertility treatment plan instead of preserving a marriage *that is not in jeopardy,* your energy will be better directed.

Internal Needs (Ego Needs)
(Statements 7–20)

Some women truly feel incomplete because of their fertility problem. Nor is it uncommon for infertile men to feel less virile.

These reactions seem to be more common among men and women from a traditional background where male and female roles are strictly defined: where the man sees himself as husband, father, and provider and the woman sees herself as wife, mother, and nurturer. Infertility obviously prevents these couples from fulfilling the primary roles they have defined for their lives.

Statements 7 through 20 will help you identify why you want or need a baby. Your answers will tell you, for example, if you want a baby so you can perpetuate your genes, so you can prove that you are virile or feminine, so you can bring meaning to your life, and/or so you can regain power over your body and destiny once more. Your motives are very important in choosing the "right" happy ending.

As you evaluate your answers to this section, you may wish to examine some of your other answers to determine (1) whether your life-style needs fit the traditional role, (2) whether you may be responding to external pressures (the needs of others) more than to your own, and (3) whether you have strong parenting and nurturing needs. I find that people who see life without children as purposeless usually *believe* that they are responding to internal needs and personal goals. In actual fact, they may be placing a higher value on their family's and society's expectations than they are on their own needs. This was the situation in Debbie's case. Debbie told me that her mother had frequently said to her, "Something's wrong with you if you don't want your own children." (See "External Pressures" below.)

If you understand the source of your motives, you will better understand the source of your discomfort and stress.

If you truly feel powerless and that life is meaningless, you may need professional counseling to help you avoid episodes of anxiety and depression. Shelley told me, "I'm certain that Michael and I are still married today because of the help we received through our RESOLVE support group."

Many of the answers in this section will help you decide which happy ending is best for *you.* Armed with this knowledge, you can design a plan with your physician that will best meet your needs.

Life-style Needs
(Statements 21–38)

Our society tends to praise and value the traditional family and frown on a childfree life-style. In reality, however, life-style needs are as valid a concern as any basic biological need.

For some the arrival of a baby makes life complete. For others the rewards of parenting will never be as satisfying as the lives they led before having a baby: lives of spontaneity, of freedom, of personal control. However, *few couples with fertility problems pause to ask themselves if they really want a baby or a pregnancy.*

A baby changes your life as much as or more than marriage itself. Baby will interrupt your sleep, your schedule, your private time, and your lovemaking. For most infertile couples the prospect of altering their lives to include a baby is a joyful goal. Planning will help smooth out the uncertainties during fertility treatment and after the new arrival.

Statements 21 through 38 will help you decide if you are *ready* to bring a baby into your life—to settle down into a different life-style—and if you are financially able to support a new family member. By comparing your answers, you'll discover whether both of you share the same life-style needs.

Bryan and Debbie got into quite a tangle when he said he wanted to continue their sailing, skiing, and traveling while she wanted to save so she could quit work and stay home with the baby: "We'd always had trouble managing our money. And if I quit, we would have to have a nest egg. After we talked about it, we decided to set aside a percentage of our income. Actually, Bryan gave up buying the sailboat he wanted and we joined a sailing club so we can rent a boat anytime we want."

Kathy's answers indicated that she wasn't ready to give up her amateur running status. "When Steven and I talked about how important my physical, competitive, and social needs were to me, he stopped bugging me about quitting. Once I was relieved of my guilt, I could proceed with an aggressive treatment program—one that eventually resulted in my pregnancy."

Compare your answers with your spouse's. Explore how your fertility treatment will affect your life-style. How will it affect your career? Your finances? Your travel? Are you willing to adjust these aspects of your life for a prolonged period of treatment? And if your fertility treatment is successful, how will the baby fit into your life?

External Pressures (The Needs of Others)
(Statements 39–62)

I find that infertile couples (as well as those who decide to remain childless) often feel that full adulthood cannot be achieved without bearing children, and that remaining childless is a sign of immaturity, selfishness, failure, and instability.

Steven's answers revealed some startling facts. Coming from a large traditional family, Steven felt that he would not truly be a man until he fathered children. Steven's dad was a very devoted family man and Steven had many fond memories of their weekends working and playing together. Steven couldn't imagine life without sons and daughters to help fill his nonworking hours. Kathy was shocked with Steven's answers: "All along I thought that Steven's 'poor' sexual performance was because he didn't really want children. When I discovered that it had to do with his self-image and not his desire for children, it shed a whole new light on our problem. One we could deal with."

Your family may exert a number of pressures on you to have a baby. Your parents may want to become grandparents. Or they may want you to continue the family lineage and name. If you seem to be overly concerned about what your family thinks and/or how to relate to them, you will be especially interested in reading chapter 20. And you may wish to show your family "A Letter to Family and Friends," which appears in the appendix.

Not having a baby makes you different—much as being single, being unemployed, or being handicapped makes you different. "Different" people must cut their own paths, define their own roles, and even defend their individuality to family, friends, and co-workers. It's little wonder that couples having fertility problems often seem driven to conquer their infertility—their "difference."

Richard and Margaret found it more and more difficult to relate to their close friends, all of whom had children. "I don't have anything in common with them," Margaret told me. "I want to talk about my most recent business trip and my girlfriend wants to talk about Andrew's preschool." Their answers to the test showed a strong need to belong—to fit into the community.

Compare how you and your spouse answer these statements. See how influenced you are by what others think. If you find you are more concerned with fulfilling the needs of your parents and society than with identifying your *own* needs, you may want to get your priorities in order.

When my patients begin to discuss how these social pressures control their emotions and actions, their decisions often turn completely around. Michael and Shelley, for example, discussed why going home for Christmas was the last thing Shelley wanted to do. "Holding my sister's new baby would be too much for me," Shelley said. "After talking it over, we gave ourselves permission to vacation in Hawaii instead."

Once my patients realize *why* outsiders have such an influence on their lives, they can handle comments from relatives, friends, and co-workers with a more positive view. And they remain true to their own convictions instead of bowing to external pressures.

Parenting and Nurturing Needs
(Statements 63–70)

This section of the test will help you explore how you feel about children. Do you want to care for them, play with them, discipline them, and teach them—for the next twenty years? For some this sounds like an awesome task; for others it sounds like a dream come true.

Not everyone enjoys diaper changing and 2:00 A.M. feedings. So if you are still ambivalent about having a baby or have doubts about your ability to care for a tiny tot, count yourself as part of the human race.

If like Margaret and Richard your answers show that you like to play with children, that you like to feed, diaper, and bathe children, and that you believe you'll make a good parent, I wouldn't worry too much about your motives for having children. These statements should confirm what you already know—that you want to love and care for a child and, perhaps most of all, you want to have fun with a family of your own.

Identifying Your Happy Ending

A fertility treatment plan should lead to a resolution that is right for you. By comparing and discussing your answers to the evaluation, you should both be well on your way toward deciding which happy endings will satisfy your emotional needs. Instead of seeing yourselves as threatened, powerless victims, you will operate as a well-coordinated team committed to common goals and a mutual plan.

It's time now to learn what your diagnostic alternatives and medical resources are for pursuing your happy ending. In the next chapter I will give you a step-by-step procedure for designing your individual fertility treatment plan.

4. How to Avoid
Hit-or-Miss Fertility Treatment

"You had surgery *before* your husband was tested?" The RESOLVE group members looked at each other in disbelief.

"Well, we thought it was *my* problem," Shelley T. said. "I've always had pain with my periods. It made sense."

"The same thing happened to us," Steven S. commented from across the room. "We thought our doctor was a specialist. That's the way he's listed in the phone directory. But when he wanted to put Kathy through a twenty-five-hundred-dollar workup and never even asked about *me*, we knew something was wrong."

"What did you do?" Shelley asked.

"We paid our fifty-dollar consultation charge and found a different doctor." Steven glanced at his wife. "One who would work with us as a couple. Infertility affects the *couple*, not just one individual."

"But how do you know if your doctor is doing the right thing?" Shelley asked.

The group leader spoke. "Learn as much about fertility problems and treatment as you can so you'll be able to ask the right questions and spot potential trouble.

"Coming to RESOLVE is the first step," he added. "You learn a lot from our programs and from talking with our members. And if you read our newsletter, you'll see that we have resource people who can talk with you about different fertility subjects—like endometriosis, artificial insemination, and in vitro fertilization. We also have an extensive lending library of books and articles on just about any fertility topic you'll want to know about."

"You mean *I'm* going to have to be responsible for my fertility treatment?"

"You *and* your husband *and* your doctor," the RESOLVE leader said. "If you work as a team, you'll be able to design a fertility treatment plan that will work for you as a couple."

The leader turned toward me. "Dr. Perloe, how *can* couples avoid hit-or-miss fertility treatment?"

"I agree with all that's been said. It's unfortunate that you cannot expect the same quality of treatment from every doctor or clinic. But I guess that's true of any kind of service." I glanced at Steven and Kathy. "I guess Steven and Kathy are one of the best prepared couples I've ever worked with. Prior to coming to me, they'd read everything they could get their hands on. Before they hired me as their doctor, they wanted to know what to expect."

Shelley interrupted. "Like what?"

"They wanted to know things like what tests I'd recommend, what the results would mean, how long the workup would take, and how much it would cost."

"Didn't you feel like they didn't trust you?"

"Not at all," I answered. "The more you know about your treatment, the better you can work with your doctor. In fact, I usually give every couple an overview of fertility treatment before we even start."

"That's right, Shelley," the leader added. "If your doctor doesn't want to answer your questions or doesn't tell you what to expect, you're probably seeing the wrong doctor. Why don't you see me after the meeting and I'll give you some of our newsletters to read."

"That sounds great," Shelley said. "And I want to see your library, too."

Beginning Your Fertility Treatment Plan

Even if you already have been through months or years of fertility treatment, it is not too late to begin a plan. Shelley and Michael T. were able to regain control once they knew what to expect and began to participate in the decisions about their treatment, and so can you.

In this chapter I'd like to acquaint you briefly with the conditions necessary for conception. And as I do with my patients, I'd like to give you an *overview* of fertility treatment. With this understanding you will be able to help your physician provide the best opportunity to reach your fertility potential.

I realize that many of the things I'll touch on will stir up more questions in your mind. However, hold your questions while I give you the *big picture*. In later chapters I'll discuss all of this information and more in greater detail.

The Eight Key Ingredients of Fertility

The goal of fertility treatment is to help you have a child. If you understand the factors necessary for making a baby, you will also understand what factors your physician will evaluate during your fertility workup. The eight key ingredients of fertility are:

1. The male must be able to produce and ejaculate functional sperm.

2. The egg must mature and escape from a woman's ovary at regular or predictable intervals.

3. The egg must be able to travel through the fallopian tubes toward the uterus.

4. A couple must have intercourse at the *right* time.

5. The sperm must be able to travel through the cervix and uterus to the fallopian tubes to join with the egg.

6. The sperm must be able to penetrate the egg.

7. The fertilized egg must be able to travel through the fallopian tube to the uterus for implantation.

8. A woman's hormone system and uterus must be able to maintain the pregnancy.

To pinpoint where things are breaking down, your physician must check out each of these eight fertility factors. Later in this book you will learn about the methods your doctor can use to investigate fertility problems and what treatment is available. When you understand your options, you will know how to get your miracle baby.

Your Fertility Workup: An Overview

Your Past Provides Important Clues

First your doctor will ask you both to complete a general health and fertility history questionnaire. Your fertility problems may be rooted in your past—exposure to toxic chemicals, medications, illnesses, and infections, for example. I remember one couple whose problem crystallized when I learned that he'd been exposed to Agent Orange in Vietnam. When I added this incident to his complaints of lethargy and low sexual desire, I began to suspect he could have a fertility problem.

Your doctor should interview you not only together but also individually so you will feel free to reveal your closest-held secrets—having had an abortion, a sexually transmitted disease, or an illegitimate child, for example. If either of you withholds information, your doctor may perform unnecessary tests and it may take longer and cost more to identify your missing fertility factors. Honesty and completeness pay off.

I remember one woman who told me in confidence about an abortion she had before she was married. Since I knew she had been fertile at that time, I began looking for events that occurred since then. When I learned she'd had a ruptured appendix at age twenty-one, I suspected the infection and surgery could have adversely affected her reproductive organs. So I began to formulate a series of tests that would give me definite answers.

Sometimes your fertility history reveals obvious problems. If like Kathy S. you have only one or two periods a year, I quickly suspect ovulatory problems. If like Shelley T. you complain of extreme pain during menstruation, I'll look for endometriosis. Or if like Margaret B. you've had one or more episodes of pelvic inflammatory disease (PID), I'll check you for tubal blockage. You will learn more about how I diagnosed and treated each of these women and their husbands later.

Some less obvious factors that can contribute to your fertility problem are:

- Previous abdominal surgeries, which may impair fertility in both men and women
- Diabetes or a case of childhood mumps, which can lead to a poor sperm count
- Drugs and high blood pressure medications, which can impair a man's sexual performance

As you are filling out your history form, you may not realize the significance of these events or conditions, but if you do your job well, your doctor will have the information he or she needs for piecing together the puzzle.

Highlights of the Male's Workup

To father a child you must be able to produce and ejaculate good quality semen. "Good" semen contains large numbers of normally formed sperm which can swim actively in a straight line. In addition, semen should be free of infection. To deliver your semen to your wife, you must also be able to ejaculate. This requires that you have open passages from your testicles to your penis and an intact nervous system for controlling your ejaculatory processes. Chapter 8 discusses all the hormonal and physiological systems necessary to support male fertility.

If the semen analysis is normal, I can be almost certain that the fertility problem lies with the woman's reproductive system. So I will switch my attention to diagnosing her problem.

If the semen analysis reveals a problem with the husband's fertility, he should have a physical examination to assess his general health and the condition of his reproductive organs. Shelley T.'s husband, Michael, had almost no sperm in his semen. I needed to find out if this was because he was not making sperm or because his sperm could not get out through his ducts.

Based on my examination findings, I may order additional tests to detect if the man has tubal blockage, impaired ejaculation, impaired sperm production, or a hormonal problem, or refer him to a urologist for further evaluation and recommendations.

Finding a fertility problem with the husband doesn't relieve my responsibility to make certain that the wife's reproductive system is working well. I find that in 20 to 30 percent of my cases, *both* partners contribute to their fertility problems. In Steven and Kathy S.'s case, for example, Steven had a poor sperm count and Kathy wasn't ovulating. Until I was fairly certain that Kathy's problem could be overcome, it would have been irresponsible for me to condone Steven's varicocoele surgery.

Chapters 6 through 8 describe in detail the tests that are conducted for male fertility problems, what the test findings reveal, and what courses of treatment are available for male fertility problems.

Highlights of the Woman's Workup

Even if a woman's periods are regular, I cannot assume that her menstrual cycle is working normally. So once I've reviewed the wife's history and current complaints, I do a physical examination to evaluate her general health and the condition of her reproductive organs. I also order laboratory tests that will tell me if she's ovulating and if her hormone levels are adequate.

I frequently include an endometrial biopsy in the initial workup because examining the uterine lining will tell me whether she's ovulating and whether her uterus can support a pregnancy. In addition, I may order an X ray to obtain valuable information on the structure of her fallopian tubes and uterus. Many of these tests must be performed at specific points in the monthly cycle. Therefore, I ask her to do some "homework" to help me time the tests.

I ask her to keep a basal body temperature (BBT) chart. This cycle will not only help me synchronize the tests to her menstrual cycle but also tell me what time of the month she is most fertile. If your temperature chart line remains level throughout the month, for example, I may suspect that you are not ovulating (anovulation). If you are timing sex *after* your temperature rises, I'll know that you are practicing rhythm *birth control,* which is certainly no way to get a miracle baby! (You are most fertile twenty-four to forty-eight hours *before* your temperature rises.)

I also perform a postcoital test to tell me if the "chemistry" between the partners is right. If the wife's cervical mucus is impairing or destroying the husband's sperm, there are a number of things I can do to improve their situation.

You will learn more about the woman's workup in chapters 9 and 10. You may even discover what's causing your fertility problem and learn how to overcome it.

The Preliminary Report

Your initial workup usually takes six to eight weeks and may cost up to $2,500. (This cost may vary in different parts of the country.) Once your doctor has the results from your examinations and preliminary tests, you can begin to discuss your options:

- Beginning a treatment program to improve your fertility
- Undergoing surgery to correct anatomical problems

- Seeking other alternatives such as artificial insemination with donor sperm (AID), in vitro fertilization, adoption, or enlisting a surrogate mother
- Performing more tests to pinpoint your fertility problem

Your doctor should outline a tentative treatment schedule as well as estimate the cost. Together you should develop a plan that will optimize your fertility while still taking into consideration your life-style needs and financial resources.

Formulating Your Treatment Plan

How Long Will It Take?

I try to give couples a treatment time frame so they know how long it may take to achieve a pregnancy. With this information they can assume more control over their time and money. For example, I told Steven and Kathy S. that if he elected to have his varicocoele repaired, it would be at least three months after the surgery before we would know if Steven's sperm count would improve. During that time Kathy could begin taking medication to induce her to ovulate. Within three months Steven's sperm count should improve and Kathy's cycle should be regulated.

Sometimes couples wonder why the workup often takes several months. Unfortunately, within one menstrual cycle we can try only a few things at a time. Since Kathy S. was not ovulating, my first priority was to induce ovulation. Once her body responded to that medication, I could then check other factors. As it turned out, I discovered a secondary problem which could prevent their fertilized egg from implanting in her uterus. So the next month I added a hormone to correct that problem.

It is for these reasons that your doctor cannot always tell you exactly how long treatment will take or how effective it will be. You do have a right to know, however, what results to expect if the procedure is a "success" or a "failure." And this knowledge will give you the tools you need to participate in the decision about what to try next.

Many people become discouraged with fertility treatment because they believe that in the first month they "become fertile" they will make a baby. We may work for four to six months regulating ovulation and improving semen quality to fertile levels. The seventh month passes—no pregnancy. The eighth month—no pregnancy. The ninth month—no pregnancy:

"I don't understand, Dr. Perloe," Margaret B. said. "We've tried everything and I'm not pregnant yet."

"Do you have friends or relatives with children?" I asked.

"Yes, my brother and sister."

"Do you know how long they tried to get pregnant?"

"Well, my brother and his wife did it in two months. But my sister took five."

"Do either of them have a fertility problem?"

"No. But why are you asking me about them?" she said.

"Well, what makes you think that you'll get pregnant within two or three months of solving your fertility problem when it took your sister—who had *no* fertility problems—five?"

She paused for a moment. "Well, I've always done everything better than my sister, and I should be able to get pregnant faster, too." She burst into a laugh.

I laughed with her. "You see my point, Margaret? Fertile people have a 20 percent chance for pregnancy each month. And people who have been through fertility treatment have at the most a 20 percent chance, too. You could easily take six months to a year to get pregnant, even if everything is in perfect working condition.

"Fertility treatment is a tremendous strain," I added. "Getting pregnant— or *not* getting pregnant—is on your mind every day. Just don't get upset about it—not yet, anyway. Remember our plan? We will try five or six cycles and then, if you aren't yet pregnant, we'll consider other options. Next time talk to me before you become upset. Okay?"

How long will treatment take? Talk to your doctor, make a plan, and monitor your progress. And don't forget that "normally fertile" people may take up to a year to get pregnant.

What Price Pregnancy?

I find that many couples are reluctant to discuss money with me because they feel guilty about placing a "price" on pregnancy or having a baby. They tend to overlook insurance and money issues when developing their fertility treatment plan.

However, fertility treatment can be quite expensive—both in actual cost and in the time you may lose from work. In fact, some treatment regimens may be so demanding that your job is placed in jeopardy. For example, certain medications must be given by injection in the doctor's office several days a week; postcoital tests require you to come in two to four hours after having sex; and diagnostic surgeries may require that you miss several days of work. It's only fair that you be aware of these requirements before committing yourself to a treatment program. Knowing what you're getting into may not change your choice, but it will give you the opportunity to plan your life and prepare your employer.

Before Michael and Shelley T. came to see me, they had had many squabbles about money. Since Michael did not understand why the tests and medications were necessary, he had no way of evaluating whether costs were getting out of hand. To make things worse, they'd bought a house, anticipating that Shelley's coming promotion would bring in more money. When Shelley's boss discovered that she'd filed insurance claims for fertility treatment, however, he promoted someone else instead. The boss *claimed* that he passed her up because she was taking three to four afternoons off per month for tests. But Shelley heard through the grapevine that he didn't want to promote her because he thought she'd probably quit after she had the baby. He also mumbled something about her medical claims increasing the company policy premiums. Although not all employers will react this way, you may have to be careful how you present your planned absenteeism and your future employment plans to your boss. I'll tell you later how other couples have handled these dilemmas.

Because this couple had not agreed upon a financially manageable treatment plan, Michael felt that he was not in control of the situation. I can understand why, when faced suddenly with a $2,000 surgical expense, they refused the doctor's recommendation for diagnostic surgery. However, if from the beginning Shelley's doctor had included Michael in the plans for her treatment, the story might have been different.

Steven and Kathy S., for example, controlled their psychological and financial resources right from the start. As a runner, Kathy's athletic achievements were very important to her. After her initial workup, I pointed out to her that her physical exertion could very well be the reason that her menstrual periods had for the most part stopped. She decided, however, that she wanted to try to keep running and achieve pregnancy, too. So together we worked out a treatment plan based on that agreement.

Since Kathy didn't work, they had a limited budget. Steven checked out what his group insurance covered before beginning treatment. The policy would pay for most expenses; however, it didn't cover everything. (Trying to keep up with what one insurance company covers and what another company doesn't is nearly impossible. The logic insurance companies use for determining eligibility is sometimes a mystery.) In the course of making their fertility treatment plan Steven and Kathy decided to begin saving for the possibility of microsurgery or in vitro fertilization, which could cost up to $5,000 or $6,000 per procedure. Even though their insurance would pay 80 percent of up to two in vitro procedures, they knew that their bill could add up to quite a bit more (many people require three or four in vitro cycles before conceiving). Since banks don't make loans for babies, they wanted to be prepared to make the right choices without facing extreme financial pressures.

It was a good thing they started their savings account, because Steven's varicocoele surgery cost $2,400. We had to make a change in the fertility plan to include using his sperm for four artificial inseminations at $400 per cycle. (Remember that this expense was in addition to Kathy's ovulation induction of about $300 per month.) And if Kathy's *oral* medication hadn't worked, she might have had to take Pergonal injections and have blood tests costing nearly $700 per month. With the Pergonal, she would also need three to five $100 ultrasound readings to monitor her egg development, a total cost of $1,000 per month. (Without ultrasound to determine the effects of the Pergonal she might risk having multiple births, and quadruplets were *not* in their plans.) I'll tell you how Kathy and Steven got their baby girl in a later chapter.

The point I'm making is that *fertility treatment can be very expensive,* and expenses may increase as you modify your fertility plan to accommodate your medical needs. Your ability to control your expenses is a vital part of your fertility plan. I suggest that you work with your doctor to estimate a best-case and worst-case scenario. That way you minimize the risk of any big surprises.

Insurance Is No Guarantee

You should talk with your doctor about the costs and with your insurance carrier about what is and is not covered. Sometimes insurance companies have riders and waiting periods before you qualify for coverage. Some policies even exclude pregnancy and fertility payments altogether. Coverage may also differ from state to state. If your company transfers you from New York Blue Cross/Blue Shield to Oklahoma Blue Cross/Blue Shield, for example, you may not have the same protection. The only way you'll know is by asking.

In addition, some fertility treatment procedures may be considered experimental and therefore will not be paid for by the insurance carrier. In vitro fertilization fit in this category for many years. Even though most companies will pay in vitro now, they often place a limit on how many cycles they will cover. You could find that an HMO (health maintenance organization offering prepaid medical care) will provide more complete coverage than standard insurance policies. Only when you have these facts and figures can you develop a treatment plan within your means.

Later chapters will tell you more about the demands of specific tests and treatment regimens as well as how couples manage their jobs, their schedules, their money, and their personal lives.

A Seven-Day-a-Week Commitment

Fertility treatment is a seven-day-a-week proposition. If you ovulate on the weekend, you may find yourself in the doctor's office having ultrasound or artificial insemination. You can't spend hundreds of dollars a month to induce ovulation and blow it because it's the Sabbath. Discuss your feelings about the time involved.

You will see how other couples handled these problems in chapter 20. In addition, I will discuss such specifics as how you can schedule a vacation while in treatment—and how you can start having fun in bed again. As a couple you need to decide how you will handle emotional issues, schedule changes, and inconveniences. *One partner cannot bear all the burden.*

Examining Your Moral and Ethical Beliefs

You also need to discuss what types of treatment plans will fit into your moral and ethical beliefs. The evaluation test in chapter 3 may have helped you analyze these issues. But once you begin formulating your treatment plan, you will have to come to grips with some heavy decisions. How do you feel about your spouse risking major surgery? Are you willing to consider artificial insemination with your husband's sperm (AIH) or with a donor's sperm (AID)? What about using a donor egg (embryo) from another woman? I'll discuss the legal and ethical implications of these and other options in chapter 21. And I'll also tell you about the decisions other couples have made.

When Will You Stop Treatment?

You should make a tentative decision about how long you will stick with one treatment approach. Although your decisions may change as you obtain more information from tests and treatments, you still should have short-term goals and concrete mileposts to measure your progress. For example, Steven and Kathy agreed to try AIH for six cycles before considering in vitro fertilization. Richard and Margaret limited themselves to three in vitro cycles. How long will you go through fertility treatment before considering adoption? Or when might you feel okay about deciding you want to remain childless?

Your decisions may be criticized by relatives and friends who don't share your sentiments. Michael and Shelley T. decided not to try AID or in vitro because of their parents' religious beliefs. I'm not sure they were totally comfortable with this turn of events, but they chose to keep peace in the family rather than be alienated.

Your Plan Isn't Carved in Stone

I find that as my patients learn more about their fertility problem, as the significance of not having children sinks in, as the treatments tax their emotional and physical health, or as their bank account dwindles, they often change their minds about what treatment they want. In addition, new options arise every year from advances made in medical research—donor embryos, laser surgery, and so forth. Many couples begin to consider options that seemed less attractive or simply were not available earlier in their treatment. For example, although Robert and Martha W. at first wouldn't even consider AID, they eventually decided that using donor sperm for artificial insemination would be better than going through in vitro fertilization procedures. They now have a beautiful, curly-haired baby girl whom they adore. Some couples decide that adoption is their best alternative. When Jamie L. dropped by my office to show me her newly adopted son, I remember her saying, "I wish now I hadn't thought of adoption as the last resort. I wouldn't trade my baby for anything."

Your plan is only a guide, a road map. At any point in the journey toward your happy ending, you can choose a different route. The chapters to come will help you become an informed consumer, so you will be able to assess all your options and take advantage of the best.

5. Finding the Right Doctor

Shelley looked toward me. "Dr. Perloe, how can couples find out which doctor to go to?"

"There are a number of alternatives. RESOLVE's list of physicians is an excellent beginning." I paused. "However, one thing that concerns me greatly is the thinking that says that *only* a fertility specialist can treat fertility problems. That simply is not true."

"But I wasted over a year going to my family doctor before I realized he was just bouncing from one thing to another," Shelley said.

"I know that can happen. But even a fertility specialist may use hit-or-miss procedures. You see, there is nothing to prevent any doctor from hanging up a shingle that says 'fertility specialist.' "

"I didn't know that," Debbie said.

"First consult with your family physician or obstetrician-gynecologist. She or he knows your medical history better than anyone. If your problem requires specialized knowledge, ask your doctor to refer you to a specialist.

"Read everything you can about fertility problems and fertility treatment. Talk to RESOLVE members and other infertile couples about their experiences and compare what's happening to you with what you learn. Talk to your doctor. Discuss your treatment plan and ask lots of questions. If it seems to you that your doctor does not have a plan, is not using 'accepted' procedures, or resents answering your questions, you may want to seek a second opinion."

"What if you don't have a doctor?" a woman across the room asked.

"Get a list of names in your area from the American Fertility Society or your local county medical society. Call or write fertility clinics for additional information. Talk to family and friends, too. Perhaps they know someone who's seeing a doctor for fertility treatment. With one in six couples in the United States seeking treatment for fertility problems, help can't be too far away. The best insurance you can have is being prepared—by reading, attending workshops, and joining support groups."

In this chapter I will tell you how to find a physician, what types of physicians or clinics to look for, and how to spot the "poor treatment" danger signs.

How to Find a Doctor

Consult Your Current Physician First

I encourage you to consult your family practice physician or obstetrician-gynecologist first. Since you've already developed a rapport, it will be easier for you to share personal and intimate facts about your sexual history and habits. Both of these physicians are trained to analyze the results from a semen analysis, blood tests, and X rays. And they know how to administer fertility treatment to both men and women. The following is a more detailed breakdown of different medical specialties.

Doctors Who Treat Fertility Problems

General Practitioner, Family Physician, Internal Medicine Specialist

Family physicians can assess your general health and investigate the potential effects of medical history, environment, and medications on your fertility. These physicians can determine if a woman is ovulating and if a man's semen is functional. Many common fertility problems may be resolved at this initial level—for example, using a basal body temperature chart to time coitus, ovulation induction, and counseling on the discontinuance of sperm-killing douches and lubricants. If your fertility problem is such that it demands it, your physician should refer you to a specialist. Since your records and test results will be provided to the specialist, you won't have wasted your money by seeing your family doctor first.

Obstetrician-Gynecologist

This physician specializes in the study and treatment of women's diseases, especially of the genitourinary and rectal tracts. In addition, he or she is concerned with the care and treatment of women during pregnancy and childbirth. Most OB-GYNs, as they are commonly called, also perform surgery. However, depending on their skills, they may or may not be able to perform microsurgery on your fallopian tubes, which is required in about 10 percent of fertility patients. Most OB-GYNs can perform a diagnostic lap-aroscopy, but if they can't do microsurgery, the laparoscopy may have to be repeated by the microsurgeon so he or she can plan your corrective surgery. OB-GYNs have access to all of the fertility diagnostic tests available, including the semen analysis. The OB-GYN should be able to treat anovulation and to perform artificial insemination.

Reproductive Endocrinology and Fertility Specialist

This is an American Board of Obstetrics and Gynecology certified subspecialty for OB-GYNs who receive extra training in endocrinology (the study of hormones) and infertility. Generally these physicians are affiliated with fertility research programs at universities, infertility clinics, or in vitro centers. They have the most up-to-date information on fertility and are skilled in microsurgery techniques.

Urologist

This physician specializes in the male genitourinary tract. The urologist can perform a semen analysis and can examine a man for a varicocoele, endocrine problems, genetic defects, or other physical abnormalities that may cause fertility problems. In addition, the urologist can perform a testicular biopsy, surgery for varicocoele repair, and vasectomy reversal.

Andrologist

This physician-scientist performs laboratory evaluations of male fertility. The andrologist need not be a medical doctor and may hold a Ph.D. degree in any number of technical areas, including microbiology, biochemistry, or andrology. Many andrologists are affiliated with fertility treatment centers and play a key role in performing in vitro fertilization.

Accept Your Physician's Referral

If you trust your doctor, you'll be inclined to trust the quality of the referral. Referral from another physician is one of the quickest and best ways to find a doctor.

Starting Your Search from Scratch

If you're faced with finding a new physician on your own, you may want to utilize some of these resources:

- *RESOLVE, Inc.* Contact your local RESOLVE, Inc., chapter or national RESOLVE, Inc., for a referral.
- *The American Fertility Society and local county medical society.* As noted, these organizations can provide you with a list of physicians who have expressed an interest in fertility treatment. Although membership in these organizations doesn't certify fertility treatment competency, this may be a good list to work from.
- *Fertility clinics.* A number of fertility clinics exist across the country. Some of them are for-profit clinics. Others are nonprofit research organizations usually associated with universities. Many of these clinics can perform your fertility workup. If not, they can provide you with a list of

physicians whom they work with in your community. Later I will discuss the different types of fertility clinics.

Should You Go to a Specialist?

Through your reading and search for information, you may have noticed that many sources recommend you avoid your family physician and obstetrician-gynecologist and go directly to a fertility specialist. I have heard couples say, "If you go to the in vitro clinic for your workup, you're getting the best." While it is certainly true that you can receive very good care through these facilities, the erroneous conclusion drawn by some couples is: "If you don't go to the in vitro center, you're settling for second best." Or even worse: "If the in vitro center can't help you, that's the final word."

You may also have heard that you can identify a fertility specialist by the fact that he or she "specializes" in fertility and *doesn't deliver babies*—the logic apparently being that if doctors are busy delivering babies, they're too busy to know enough about fertility to practice it. I don't believe this is an adequate description, however, of a physician who is qualified to treat your fertility problem. So for a number of reasons, which I'll share with you, I disagree with this generalized recommendation for fertility specialists.

Any physician can be listed as a fertility specialist. There is no regulation, licensing, or certification required for advertising this specialty. Before you make your first appointment, however, you can inquire if the physician is *board-certified* in the reproductive endocrinology and infertility subspecialty. To become board-certified, the physician must meet educational requirements and pass written tests.

Membership in the American Fertility Society is available to any physician showing an interest in the specialty. While membership in this organization does not guarantee a known standard of technical competence, it does demonstrate the physician's interest in fertility treatment (a definite plus).

Specialists may charge more for the same services. An article in *Money* magazine stated that fertility specialists may charge up to five times more than nonspecialists. This may be overstated, but before you settle on the physician you want, ask about the charges for common tests and procedures. You may find that you'll pay twenty to twenty-five dollars more for a semen analysis from a specialist, even though the same medical laboratory provides these services to all of the doctors in your community. Do a little price comparison first and remember that the lowest- or highest-priced doctor is not necessarily the worst or best.

The Private Physician vs. the Fertility Clinic

Another question that arises is whether to consult with a private physician or go to a large fertility clinic. A private physician can treat most fertility problems. The additional skills and expertise provided by in vitro centers and large fertility clinics are needed only for about 10 percent of fertility problems. I have some additional ideas on this matter that I'd like to share with you:

For-profit fertility clinics and in vitro centers are not certified and their reported results aren't validated. Fertility treatment has become a big moneymaking business. It's little wonder that the clinic's interest in attracting customers influences the way in which they may report their pregnancy success rates. For example, a clinic may report that 25 percent of their patients get pregnant within three cycles. So you may assume that you have a one in four chance of pregnancy if you go to them. These could look like pretty good odds to some couples. However, the clinic's statistics do not show that they eliminate more than half of the applicants before attempting any in vitro procedures. So in actual fact only 25 percent of the remaining half of their patients (or really 12.5 percent of *all* their patients) actually succeed. Don't get me wrong: Many of these clinics are quite reputable and do show impressive results. Just try to be objective when you read or hear about their services and success rates.

Research-oriented clinics may perform unnecessary tests and procedures to meet research criteria and to pay their expenses. In order to conduct scientifically sound fertility research, medical professionals must have similar information about each couple. Thus this kind of clinic may perform expensive tests not only on patients who warrant them but also on those who do not need them. In this way the researchers can compare their results between "abnormal" and "normal" populations. Consequently the research clinic may not tailor your workup to your unique set of problems. Money charged for these "extra" tests also helps pay the bills for expensive laboratory and research capabilities which may not be needed for your basic diagnostic workup. Before signing up with a research clinic, find out what diagnostic procedures they recommend and how much they charge. If this information doesn't correlate with what you've learned about fertility treatment, you may wish to get a second opinion.

Larger clinics may contribute to your feeling of isolation and anonymity. Often couples who have gone to large clinics complain that they didn't receive much of the physician's personal time; no one in the clinic knew them by sight; and a different resident physician saw them at each visit. Also, many people who travel considerable distances to these clinics don't feel comfortable expressing their concerns: they feel isolated and dissatisfied. One patient said, "I feel like I'm being herded like cattle." If that's the way you feel, you probably are not getting the personal attention you need, and the clinic you're going to may be too large. I must say, however, that a number of large clinics provide services that many smaller organizations cannot: educational videotapes, nurse practitioners to answer questions, on-site X-ray and testing laboratories, and counseling and support groups—all of which can be of great value.

For-profit fertility clinics tend to charge more for basic diagnostic workups and treatments than do family practitioners and obstetrician-gynecologists. I find that people who go to fertility and in vitro clinics for standard workups and treatment tend to pay *50 to 100 percent more* than those going to private practitioners. These charges result in part from the higher overhead these clinics incur for elaborate testing, surgical, and research facilities. You may be paying for testing and treatment capabilities that you don't need for your basic diagnostic workup. Find out what they charge and compare their rates to what other doctors charge in your community.

Many communities are not large enough to support fertility specialists and in vitro clinics. Traveling to distant medical facilities may add unnecessarily to your out-of-pocket expenses, absenteeism from work, and overall level of stress. If you have a good family practitioner and/or OB-GYN in your community who knows quite a bit about fertility treatment, I'd encourage you to begin there rather than travel hundreds of miles to a stranger. The "expert" isn't necessarily better just because he or she is located over one hundred miles away.

A Final Note About Selecting a Doctor

Fertility treatment isn't magic. It is a structured, organized investigation. An obstetrician-gynecologist working together with a urologist can diagnose and successfully treat the majority of people with fertility problems.

Ultimately you should judge any doctor's ability based on the treatment plan he or she outlines especially for you and on the doctor's responsiveness to your problems and concerns.

Making a List and Checking It Twice

The first interview with your doctor provides an excellent opportunity for you to assess how well you will be able to work together.

To prepare for your first visit, write down a list of questions you want to ask. To help formulate your questions, you may want to refer to the workup overview in chapter 4 as well as to the next section, which lists the questions people most frequently ask me. The reasons for asking some of these questions may not make complete sense until you've read the rest of this book. However, I feel I should put them here so you have them as background.

If you are already receiving fertility treatment, it is not too late to ask your doctor these questions. If you spot any of the "Four Poor Treatment Danger Signs" discussed below, you may wish to reconsider your choice of doctors.

Questions to Ask Your Doctor

About the Doctor's Practice

Do you have experience in fertility treatment?

Will you refer me to an obstetrician when I get pregnant or will you deliver the baby?

Will you send me to any other physicians or laboratories for treatments or tests?

Will you treat my spouse? If not, who will?

Do you arrange for adoptions?

Do you document surgeries with photographs or videotapes so I can see your findings for myself or provide them to other doctors?

Which hospital(s) do you use?

Do you use Pergonal to induce ovulation? If so, do you monitor egg development with ultrasound to avoid multiple births?

Do you perform sterilization reversals? What is your success rate? (Should be about 50 percent.)

Do you perform microsurgery? What is your success rate for vasectomy reversal? (Should be about 90 percent.) For fallopian tube repair? (Should be 50 to 70 percent.)

Do you belong to the American Fertility Society?

Are you on the RESOLVE, Inc., recommended list of physicians?

About Tests, Surgery, and Treatments

What kind of procedure is it?

What will the procedure tell you?

What results do you expect?

How long will it take?

What will it cost? Does insurance cover it?

Will it hurt?

How will it make me feel afterward?

Can you do it in your office? As a hospital outpatient?

Will I be incapacitated? For how long? Will I miss work?

Will my spouse be involved? How? Will he/she miss work?

Can I drive home afterward?

How many times will it be repeated?

Will it interfere with our sex life? How?

Will we have to delay our vacation?

About Medications

What results do you expect?

How long/often will I take it?

What will it cost? Does insurance cover it?

Will it hurt or have side effects?
Do I take it at home or at your office?
Will I have to miss time at work?
How many times will it be repeated?
Will we have to delay our vacation?

Four Poor Treatment Danger Signs

Once you've selected your physician, *you are responsible for monitoring your doctor's performance.* That may sound strange to you, but if you hired a carpenter, auto mechanic, or roofer, you wouldn't think twice about making sure you were getting the work you contracted for. It's the same for a doctor. However, you must be an informed consumer in order to evaluate the doctor's performance.

Below are four danger signs that will alert you that you may have chosen the wrong person:

1. *No clear-cut fertility treatment plan.* If your physician does not formulate and discuss a treatment plan, you may be on the "hit-or-miss" regimen. After your first conference, your doctor should be able to outline the initial phases of your workup. After the basic workup, which may take four to six weeks, your doctor should be able to outline a treatment plan. You should be confident that your doctor, as would any good investigator, is using specific step-by-step procedures for getting answers about your fertility problem. If your doctor hasn't shared the plan with you, ask for a detailed explanation. (I'll describe the nature of these plans later.)

Take notes and make sure that your doctor follows that course. If your doctor deviates from the plan, find out why. Was it because of an unexpected test result? Or did the doctor forget certain details that were planned initially? Remember, *ask questions when they arise.* Waiting for the straw that breaks the camel's back or assuming that the doctor is an infallible being who will take care of everything will get you into trouble. If your doctor's response to your request for a plan is not adequate, find a different doctor.

2. *Poor communication.* If you can't talk to your doctor, at least one of you has a problem. Doctors are usually very busy, so as a rule they won't sit down and strike up a conversation hoping that eventually you will feel at ease enough to ask a question. If, after you leave the doctor's office, you always remember a question you meant to ask, I encourage you to write down your questions before your appointments. You should feel free to call back and talk to the nurse practitioner or to the doctor personally. If you feel that your doctor is not taking your questions seriously, is giving you superficial answers, seems impatient about explaining terms and treatment, persistently talks over your head, will not return your calls, or is too frequently not available when you need help, find another.

3. *Unorthodox treatment or methods.* After reading this book, you will be well acquainted with the methods your doctor should be using. If your doctor deviates from these regimens—for example, by failing to perform a semen analysis, prescribing fertility drugs before doing a complete fertility evaluation, or administering Pergonal without using an ultrasound to monitor the number of eggs you're developing—you have reason to be concerned.

Talk to your physician. Don't just assume he or she is incompetent. You may have misunderstood something you heard or read, or your condition might be out of the ordinary. If after getting the doctor's answers you are still troubled, however, you may wish to request a second opinion, especially when surgery is recommended. No good doctor should balk at this perfectly reasonable request. If you don't think your doctor is using the "best" fertility treatment procedures or if you lack faith in your doctor's decisions, then find another doctor.

4. *Your treatment is taking too long.* This is a tough one because the amount of time required to diagnose and treat each fertility problem is different for each patient. However, there are a few benchmarks you can watch for. Your initial workup should be complete within four to six weeks—two months at the most. At that point your doctor should be able to give you the preliminary findings and should present your options for additional tests or treatment.

As your treatment progresses, you may tend to become impatient. You may forget, for example, that even after you are "cured," you are no more fertile than the average population at your age. At the most, you have a 20 percent chance of getting pregnant each month. So if your doctor feels that your fertility problem is resolved after six months of treatment, it may take another six to nine months for you to get pregnant. If you don't conceive in that time, your doctor may recommend conducting further tests.

Doctors may often use a more aggressive treatment approach with an older couple like Richard and Margaret B., who were in their mid-thirties. A woman in that age group doesn't have that many fertile years left and her odds for "normal" pregnancy are getting slimmer each year. If you feel your fertile years are slipping away, discuss your concerns with your doctor. If your doctor isn't responsive, find another doctor.

I tailor the rate of treatment to each couple. Some people want to know all of the answers *right now.* Others want to proceed more slowly—they need time for things to sink in. For example, Shelley T. had a limited budget, so the pacing of her treatment plan was slower than for Margaret, who wanted to get pregnant as soon as possible. Each of these women required a custom-designed treatment plan that would accommodate her life-style.

Is your treatment taking too long? That's very hard to judge. But if you're really worried about it, talk with your doctor and your RESOLVE support group counselors. *If you don't feel that you're making progress, get a second opinion or find a new doctor.*

I encourage you to learn as much as you can about fertility treatment and, above all, never to accept your doctor's recommendations complacently. Ultimately *you* are responsible for the quality of care you receive. You are responsible for selecting the doctor who is best qualified to help you get your miracle baby.

II. Male Fertility

6. The Formula for Male Fertility

The day that Michael T. heard that he had no sperm in his semen, he almost stormed out of my office. Hearing the news didn't do much for Shelley either:

"A year of tests for nothing!" she said.

"Don't be so hasty. They weren't exactly for *nothing*," I assured her. "You did find out you have endometriosis, which impairs your fertility. Only now we know that we must treat *both* of you. You may have that baby yet."

Many couples overreact to the results of a single semen analysis, just as Michael and Shelley T. did. However, since many factors can "spoil" or influence a single test result—errors in collection, errors in handling the specimen, and errors at the laboratory—I always advise performing a second semen analysis in a month or so. Convincing Michael and Shelley of this wasn't easy.

"The semen analysis is only a screening test," I explained. "It does not provide a definitive diagnosis. It tells me the quality and quantity of your sperm, the motility or movement of your sperm, the volume of your semen, and the concentration of your sperm. In plain English it tells me if you are producing the right amount of good quality sperm *and* semen."

"What did my test show?"

"I found almost no sperm and very little semen or fluid. This can mean a number of things: You do not produce much semen and sperm. You produce semen and sperm but due to an obstruction they do not come out when you ejaculate. Or, perhaps even more simply, you didn't collect the sample correctly. That's what I need to find out first."

Semen Analysis

If the semen analysis establishes that the man is fertile and free from infection, no further fertility testing will be needed of him. The only remaining factor that might impair his sperm is incompatibility between his semen and his wife's cervical mucus. This can be checked in a postcoital test which I'll describe. However, if his semen analysis indicates a fertility problem, further evaluation is necessary.

Collecting the Semen Sample

Before I could evaluate the validity of Michael's semen analysis results, I needed to find out how he and Shelley had collected the sample. (To collect semen, a man must ejaculate into a sterile jar.) I asked them these questions:

"When you collected the sample, how long had it been since the last time you ejaculated?" Each ejaculation affects your sperm supply, so specimen collection timing should be as close to your normal ejaculation frequency as practical. (When figuring this interval, you need to consider both sex and masturbation.) Having this information is vital for correctly interpreting semen analysis findings. For example, if you ejaculate infrequently, your sample will contain a higher than expected number of dead sperm and sloughed-off cells. If you ejaculate very frequently (for example, once a day), you may not have time to replenish your sperm supply between emissions. Altering your normal pattern just to perform the test—either sooner or later—can distort the results. Michael reported that he produced the specimen at his normal frequency of ejaculation.

"How long did it take you to get the specimen to our laboratory for testing?" Normally I suggest collection at our laboratory site in our specially prepared soundproof room. However, a number of men have difficulty masturbating on demand in the doctor's office. It's at best embarrassing, and some even refuse for moral and religious reasons. I try to circumvent these obstacles as best as possible without seriously jeopardizing the integrity of the test. If the specimen is collected at home and delivered within one hour, we should be able to evaluate sperm quality. If the "home" results are abnormal, the test must be repeated to determine whether the sample was damaged in transit. If the couple wishes, the wife can help with the collection.

Using on-site facilities ensures that you collect the sample in a sterile container, that you do not expose your sample to temperatures above 70 degrees Fahrenheit, and that your sperm don't deteriorate from remaining in seminal plasma for more than half an hour. By testing your sample immediately, we can also examine how it changes consistency. Normally your semen coagulates after ejaculation to prevent spillage. It should begin to liquefy within twenty minutes to one hour. If the semen remains coagulated, it traps your sperm and prevents them from swimming to the egg. Once identified, I can easily solve coagulation problems.

Michael assured me that he had brought the specimen to the office within an hour: "Your nurse suggested that since we live so far away we get a motel room down the street. You should have seen the motel clerk," Michael said, "when they saw we had no luggage."

"How did you collect the sample, and did you save the entire ejaculation?" The best way to collect your semen is by masturbating into a sterile wide-mouth jar. I don't recommend using jars washed in a dishwasher, since they contain harmful soap residue. It's extremely important that you collect the entire specimen because the concentration of sperm varies in different portions of your ejaculate. For 90 percent of the male population, the first squirt (ejaculate fraction) contains more sperm than later portions. Subsequent squirts contain primarily semen (seminal vesicle secretions). For these reasons, you cannot collect a good sample by withdrawing your penis during sex and taking a sample of remaining squirts. You cannot withdraw in time to save the first drop of sperm-rich semen.

Since Michael T.'s religious beliefs forbade masturbation (that's actually why he refused testing with their previous doctor), I provided him with a Mylex pouch to fit around his penis during sex. I cautioned him not to use a condom or lubricants, since they often contain sperm-killing chemicals. Although Shelley complained of some discomfort with the loose-fitting plastic pouch, they both found this procedure more acceptable and were able to collect a complete sample. Where religious beliefs forbid the use of contraceptive devices, inserting a small hole near the top of the collection pouch will satisfy the patient's objections and provide an adequate specimen.

Substituting the Postcoital Examination

If a man is unable or unwilling to collect a semen sample, I can examine the wife's cervical mucus several hours after unprotected intercourse. If I find living, mobile sperm, the chances of the man's being fertile are pretty good. Under ordinary circumstances, however, the postcoital test does not give me as much information as the semen analysis, because I cannot evaluate the percentage of deformed sperm or take a white blood cell count to test for infection.

Repeating the Semen Analysis

"Michael, I feel pretty confident that the results of your semen analysis are correct. However, I want you to repeat the test in four to six weeks.

"I never jump to conclusions from a single negative test result. And you shouldn't either. Too many things can influence the results." I glanced at his medical history form. "I see you're diabetic. I want to do a physical on you and also evaluate your hormones. You aren't down for the count yet. You and Shelley have many options we haven't even discussed."

I closed his file and leaned back in my chair. "I frequently find a condition called retrograde ejaculation in diabetics. It's possible that your bladder sphincter muscle, which normally directs your semen out through your penis, is not closing. Your sperm may be squirting back into your bladder instead."

"Can you do something for it?" Shelley asked hopefully.

"Yes. But first, we need to find out exactly what we're dealing with."

"Okay, let's do it." Michael turned toward Shelley and said, "We'd better reserve that motel room again."

What Is Semen Quality?

To fertilize an egg (ovum), your sperm must be able to perform these critical tasks:

- Your sperm must be able to swim to the egg with a vigorous straight motion (motility, forward progression).
- Your sperm must be able to penetrate the egg to deliver your genes for fertilization (sperm penetration).

The semen analysis tells me if your sperm meet the first criteria. The sperm penetration assay (hamster test) or acrosin test will tell me if your sperm can penetrate the egg for fertilization. I'll discuss egg penetration tests in later chapters.

Sperm Count

American Fertility Society guidelines say a normal sperm count consists of 50 million sperm per ejaculate with 50 percent motility and 60 percent normal morphology (form). We know that concentrations must be under 20 million sperm per milliliter of ejaculate in order to actually impair fertility. Provided your sperm show adequate forward motility and good egg penetration, concentrations as low as 5 to 10 million can produce a pregnancy.

It's interesting to note that only twenty-five years ago counts of 100 million sperm per ejaculate were the norm. With time, the effects of our toxic environment and/or life-style seem to be gradually degrading male sperm counts.

Low Semen Volume

Your total semen volume also influences your fertility. If the volume is too small, say under one milliliter, you may not have enough fluid to bring the sperm in contact with your wife's cervix (the entrance of her womb). In addition, an insufficient quality of protective semen will expose your sperm to the acid, sperm-killing environment of her vagina. I remember one couple who had been trying to have a baby for over three years. When I checked the husband's semen, I found a low semen volume and a depressed sugar (fructose) level. Since the seminal vesicles (glands that produce most of the seminal fluid) produce this sugar, I suspected an obstruction or infection. When I examined him further, I found evidence of infection. After several rounds of antibiotics, his semen volume doubled to normal levels. When semen volume cannot be increased, artificial insemination (AIH) provides excellent results by delivering concentrated sperm to the womb.

High Semen Volume

If your ejaculate averages more than 3.5 milliliters, your sperm concentration may be too low; that is, your sperm are diluted by excess seminal fluid. We know that for 90 percent of men, the first portion of their ejaculate is richest in sperm. So if you produce too much semen, I'll suggest that you and your wife use coitus interruptus during sex. By withdrawing your penis from your wife's vagina after the first squirt, you can avoid diluting the mixture with subsequent squirts. This technique often yields good results as measured by a postcoital test. If "natural" means don't work, you can collect a split ejaculate by masturbating into two different containers. I can then use the sample with the highest sperm concentration for AIH.

Semen Viscosity

Semen viscosity (liquid flow) also affects your fertility potential. If your coagulated semen does not liquefy within an hour of ejaculation, your sperm may be trapped in the cottage cheese–like jelly. I remember one man whose semen did not liquefy. Since the prostate gland secretes the chemical required for liquefication, I did a rectal examination to check his gland. He just about jumped off the table when I pressed on the swollen tissue. Fortunately his infected prostate responded to antibiotic therapy.

The most common way of dealing with persistent coagulation or high viscosity is collecting your sperm through masturbation, washing the semen from them, and using your sperm for artificial insemination (AIH). I'll discuss these procedures in more detail.

Sperm Agglutination

A microscopic examination will tell me if your sperm are clumping together (agglutinating). I've seen a number of semen samples where the sperm orient themselves tail-to-tail or head-to-head instead of swimming in a straight line. This clumping prevents them from swimming to the egg. This finding may indicate a problem with sperm antibodies or the presence of a bacterial infection. I'll discuss how we can solve these problems.

Sperm Morphology

A normal-looking sperm has an oval head and a tail seven to fifteen times longer than the head. You can identify defective sperm by their large heads or strange tails—kinked, doubled, or coiled. The American Fertility Society says good quality semen should contain 60 percent normal sperm morphology. (See figure 6-1.)

The reason all men produce abnormal sperm (up to 40 percent) is not known. However, considering the rate at which your production line operates—ten million to fifty million new sperm per *day*—some attrition should be expected. We do know that toxins such as lead have been linked to reduced motility; organic solvents to coiled tails; and excessive scrotal heat to coiled tails in animal sperm. When you lower your exposure to these agents, abnormal morphology levels usually decrease. I remember one man who transferred to a different job at his company so he could avoid exposure to heat from a blast furnace. Within a few months his sperm motility and morphology showed definite improvement.

Debris and Infection

Too many underdeveloped or *immature sperm* (germinal cells) in your semen indicate *testicular stress* from illness or infection. I remember one young athlete who had recently recovered from a case of the flu where he'd run a 104-degree temperature for three days straight. His sperm count, revealing many dead and immotile sperm, nearly blew his mind. "Don't worry," I told him. "Your fever probably caused all the damage." I retested him three months later and found him fully recovered.

If I find *white blood cells* (leukocytes) in your semen, I suspect an infection. I will want to check both you and your wife for infection, since these diseases are easily passed back and forth between sexual partners. Sexually transmitted infections such as gonorrhea and ureaplasma respond to doxycycline, a tetracycline derivative. Prostate infections, which can be especially stubborn to treat, may take a month or more to clear up.

Asthenospermia (Low Sperm Motility) with Adequate Concentration and Morphology

Low motility may be a sign of infection or exposure to toxic substances. If your semen contains white blood cells and other cellular debris, you probably have an infection, which should respond well to antibiotic therapy. I will also ask if you are using medications or "street" drugs like marijuana, which can impair sperm motility. Changing medications or stopping drug usage will usually improve motility. Low motility is also quite common in the presence of a varicocoele. If other causes have been eliminated, I may recommend that

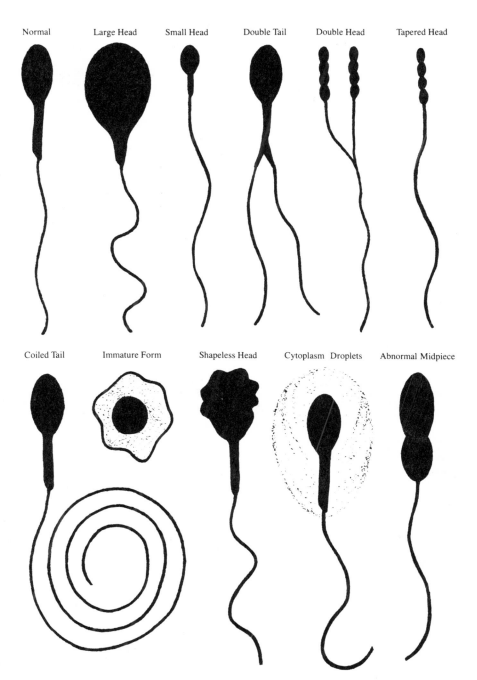

Figure 6-1. Sperm Morphology

the varicose vein be repaired. Nearly half of the men who have this surgery impregnate their wives.

If I find small testicles, scanty pubic hair, or a thinning beard, I will run blood tests to confirm a hormonal deficiency. Chapter 8 discusses when varicocoele repair or hormone replacement therapy is a waste of time and money and when it will work wonders.

Sperm-Mucus Interaction (the Postcoital Test)

Your sperm must be able to survive their journey through your wife's reproductive system. The first barriers your sperm encounter are her highly acidic vaginal fluids and cervical mucus. The vaginal environment does a good job of keeping bacteria under control, so in that way it's beneficial. However, the sperm must be specially equipped to make the journey intact. The postcoital test will tell me if your sperm are getting to your wife's uterus in good shape and in adequate numbers.

I perform the postcoital test near the middle of your wife's monthly cycle (when she should be most fertile). At the time of ovulation her cervical mucus, which normally seals her womb from the outside, becomes thin and watery to allow your sperm to swim through the cervix toward her waiting egg. If the test is done at the "wrong" time of her cycle, the results will be abnormal, since before and after ovulation the mucus becomes impervious to sperm. This is why I repeat the test every other day until her basal body temperature (BBT) rises, indicating that she has ovulated.

When I examine her cervical mucus within two or three hours after sex, I look for three things: (1) if you delivered good quantities of sperm to her cervix, (2) if your sperm are vigorously swimming through the mucus in one direction, and (3) if white blood cells are present, indicating infection in either partner. Assuming your semen analysis was normal, if I find immotile, clumped, or dead sperm in the mucus, I'll suspect that your sperm and your wife's mucus are incompatible. If I find no sperm at all, I may suspect a problem with the way you're having sex.

Even though the postcoital test provides very valuable information, I cannot substitute this test for a semen analysis, which gives me a better picture of morphology and the presence of infection (white blood cell count).

Normal Semen Analysis with Poor Postcoital Test

If I find *no* sperm in the cervical mucus, as I did with Michael and Shelley T., I suspect a delivery problem. Perhaps the husband is ejaculating prematurely and not depositing the sperm near the cervix. Maybe he is not actually ejaculating at all. Or maybe she is douching immediately after sex. I can often identify the problem by talking with the couple.

I remember one man who had a great sperm count but no sperm at all showed up in their postcoital test. After counseling with him, I discovered that when he had sex he faked his climax and did not ejaculate. After several months of counseling (costing far less than fertility treatment), he and his wife returned for another postcoital evaluation and all looked well. "It's only a matter of time now," I told them. "Just let nature take its course."

If I find agglutinated (coagulated) semen that contains shaking sperm instead of actively swimming sperm, I suspect that something in the mucus is attacking the sperm. Vaginal lubricants or allergic responses to the sperm can also cause this toxic reaction; for example, the woman's immune system may be producing antibodies that are attacking the sperm. In some situations the man himself may be making antibodies in his own sperm. I find this among men with frequent genital infections and with men who have undergone a vasectomy reversal.

Overcoming Sperm Antibodies

Using a condom during sex can sometimes reduce a wife's sensitivity to her husband's sperm. If she avoids all contact with her husband's sperm—her hands, her mouth, her genitals, and so forth—for three months or so, her antibodies may decrease in numbers. A repeat postcoital test at three-month intervals will tell me if this procedure is working. Once her antibodies stop attacking his sperm, they can swim to her egg and make a baby.

Some people do not want to wait as long as a year for the *possibility* that her antibodies will decrease. So usually I use artificial insemination with the husband's sperm to bypass sperm-mucus interaction problems. This is the route Steven and Kathy S. eventually took. AIH often works quite well. I will discuss these procedures in greater detail in chapter 21.

Concentrating Your Sperm

Sometimes I can improve the quality of your semen without having to diagnose and treat an underlying fertility problem. Concentrating your sperm by natural means or in the laboratory may improve your semen quality enough so that your wife can get pregnant without expensive medications and surgeries.

The "Natural" Split Ejaculate

When you climax, you usually ejaculate several times. You can concentrate your semen naturally by withdrawing your penis from your wife's vagina after your first sperm-rich squirt. Frequently the withdrawal–split-ejaculate technique works quite well.

AIH with the Split Ejaculate

If the "natural" split-ejaculate technique fails, I can boost your odds a bit by having you collect a split-ejaculate specimen for artificial insemination (AIH). This is also an effective way to treat infertility in men who produce low quantities of sperm. When I use the split-ejaculate method, I always examine both semen fractions, because 10 percent of men have the highest concentration of sperm in later portions. I wouldn't want to throw out the good stuff by mistake.

Centrifuging Semen for AIH

Centrifuging your semen and using the more concentrated portion for AIH may also improve your semen quality. Sometimes this technique is used with in vitro procedures.

Freezing Multiple Semen Samples for AIH

Unfortunately, collecting and freezing several sperm samples will not increase sperm quantity and concentration. The freezing and thawing processes damage the sperm so severely that semen quality actually diminishes. It's interesting, however, that sperm from a fertile donor does not deteriorate from freezing as much as that from an infertile donor.

If sperm concentration techniques do not work, I have to look for underlying causes. Chapters 7 and 8 explain how I can identify the causes of your problem and outline a fertility treatment plan.

Hit-or-Miss Male Fertility Treatment

In the past the understanding and treatment of male fertility lagged far behind that of female fertility. Infertile men were treated *empirically*. Without ever undergoing a thorough diagnosis, most men received a random series of treatments.

Many times I've heard my patients say, "I had a low sperm count, so the doctor gave me Serophene. He said if that didn't work, we'd try Pergonal." When I asked them if their doctor ran tests to find out *why* the sperm count was low, more often than not they said no. This type of treatment consumes a lot of precious time as well as your energy and money. Therefore, you should insist on getting an accurate diagnosis and treatment for a *known problem*.

Evaluating male fertility can be time-consuming and frustrating because sperm take approximately ninety days to form and mature. So if your doctor does something today to enhance your sperm production, it may be ninety days before the improved sperm show up in your semen sample.

With the advent of in vitro fertilization techniques, we're seeing rapid advances in male fertility diagnosis and treatment. Doctors now know how to *direct* therapy to the source of your problem. Today we can correctly diagnose 80 percent of our male fertility patients. And we can successfully treat over half of those. These results are pretty impressive when you consider the aim—the creation of a new human life.

7. Evaluating Male Fertility

"Dr. Perloe," Steven S. said as he sat down on the examining table, "this may sound like a dumb question, but how can I be infertile? I thought people like that wouldn't be able to 'get it up.' "

I smiled. "That's not a dumb question at all. But 'getting *it up*' and getting *them out* are two different things." I sat on the stool beside the table.

Steven still looked anxious. "You mean you can have one problem without the other?"

"Yes, you can have a completely normal sex drive and still not make enough sperm to get your wife pregnant."

"What a relief." He relaxed and the tension left his face. "I almost didn't have the courage to ask you."

"Please don't ever feel that way, Steven." I picked up his completed medical history form. "Let's see what we can do to raise your sperm count."

Steven's concern about virility is common among men. Although we see a connection between virility and fertility with a few hormonal disorders, sexual impairment is fairly rare.

In this chapter you will discover how your life-style, general health, and sexual experiences may be affecting your fertility. And you'll learn more about how your doctor can identify the source of your fertility problem.

The Four Factors of Male Fertility

To get your wife pregnant, you must be able to make and ejaculate viable sperm. To accomplish this, a number of mechanisms must be in good working order. I divide my *fertility formula* into the following categories: pretesticular, testicular, posttesticular, and ejaculatory processes. The interruption of any one of these four processes accounts for about 80 percent of male fertility problems. The other 15 to 20 percent are very rare conditions or disorders that cannot be diagnosed at this time.

Before covering each of the fertility formula factors in depth, I'd like to give you an overview of the four processes. In the next two chapters I'll discuss these areas in greater detail.

Pretesticular Function (Hormones)

Disturbances in the hormonal system cause about 10 percent of male fertility problems.

Your brain plays a key role in regulating the hormones that affect the development of sperm (spermatogenesis). The process begins when your hypothalamus (a part of your brain) emits a substance (gonadotropin-releasing hormone, or GnRH) that stimulates your pituitary gland, located at the base of your brain. Your pituitary gland then emits LH (luteinizing hormone) and FSH (follicle-stimulating hormone). These stimulate testicular development and sperm production. LH also initiates the testicular production of testosterone—a hormone responsible for virility, male secondary sex characteristics, and the support of sperm production. (If you got through that, the rest will be a cinch!)

A number of conditions can interfere with the development and timely delivery of these hormones. When the system breaks down, low sperm production (oligospermia) or no sperm production (azospermia) may result. If you have a pretesticular problem, you have a good chance of responding to hormone replacement therapy.

Testicular Function

Testicular failure represents about 55 percent of male fertility problems.

To respond to hormone stimulation properly, your testicles, or testes, must be capable of producing sperm (spermatogenesis). To assess your testicular potential, I need to know if your testes descended into your scrotum on time; if they have been damaged by a varicocoele (a varicose vein in the scrotum) or by excessive heat, toxins, disease, or trauma; or if for some genetic reason they failed to develop normally. If the damage or failure is severe, nothing much can be done to improve testicular performance. However, testes damaged by varicocoeles (which are found in 40 percent of men with fertility problems) frequently respond to surgical repair. And testes impaired by toxic substances often recover when the toxins are removed.

Posttesticular Function

Tubal obstruction—including vasectomy—accounts for about 6 percent of male infertility.

Your posttesticular system of ducts must be capable of storing and delivering your sperm. Sperm delivery system problems include obstruction or interruption of the tubes as a result of congenital malformation, disease, surgery, or trauma. Laser surgery and microsurgical techniques offer excellent chances for duct repair and restored fertility.

Ejaculatory Disturbances, Impotence, and Sexual Problems

Ejaculatory disturbances, impotence, and sexual problems may prevent you from delivering sperm to your wife's vagina. These disorders represent about 10 percent of male fertility problems.

Premature ejaculation, delayed ejaculation, and impotence may stem from surgery, medication, or physiological disturbances which respond well to hormone replacement therapy. Altering sex techniques and counseling often overcome psychologically based sexual performance difficulties.

Making the Diagnosis Is Not Always Easy

Fitting you neatly into one of these categories is not always easy. Sometimes a man will have mild or moderate symptoms or he will have several different problems, so complaints and test results will appear confusing or in conflict. For these reasons, *I caution my patients not to jump to conclusions from preliminary test results and not to attempt self-diagnosis*. If you have a fertility problem, the only way you can get an accurate diagnosis is to have a complete fertility workup, combined with careful analysis by a professional.

Clues from Your Past:
Analyzing Your Life-style

Many people suspect that doctors never read those long complicated history forms you fill out. This isn't true, especially with fertility evaluations. Your general medical history, life-style, and current symptoms provide vital clues that help your doctor pinpoint potential difficulties.

Travel, Work, Hobbies, and Activities

We know that certain chemicals can adversely affect sperm development (spermatogenesis) and lower sperm counts. Since Steven S. had a low count (oligospermia), I wanted to find out if he had ever come in contact with *toxic chemicals* like lead, pesticides, polystyrene, xylene, benzene, mercury, Agent Orange, anesthetic gases, and solvents. Long-term exposure to these chemicals can cause irreversible damage; however, removing the toxin can often restore fertility.

One unusual case surfaced a couple of years ago when a thirty-two-year-old chemical technician with oligospermia was referred to me by his company doctor. When I questioned Paul W., I discovered that several times each day he used various chemical solutions to clean metal parts. He told me that he often didn't use his safety mask because he couldn't see well with it on. After I talked to the company safety director about the composition of the cleaner, I advised Paul that some of the chemicals he used had been linked to depressed sperm production. "Either use the mask or find another job," I told him. I guess he took me seriously, because without any further treatment I found a marked regeneration of sperm three months later. Before the year was out, his wife was pregnant.

Accidental and medically prescribed exposure to large amounts of *radiation* to the gonads (to combat a malignant tumor, for example) can also impair sperm production. If your tissue damage is not extensive, however, some degree of fertility may regenerate. (*Note:* Normal, diagnostic X-ray studies do not impair fertility.)

We also know that *excessive exposure to heat* can interfere with sperm production. One reason that your sperm-producing testicles are located in your scrotum is to lower their temperature one or two degrees below your body's. I remember one man I treated who worked out at the gym four times a week and afterward soaked in the 106-degree whirlpool. His biceps were bigger than my thighs. When I found his low sperm count, I asked him to give up the whirlpool. Several months later I received a phone call from him saying his wife was pregnant.

Some jobs may overheat your scrotum (from the temperature, not from your boss breathing down your neck)—for example, the foundry worker or the sedentary long-distance truck driver. Oligospermia in the wheelchair-bound paraplegic also may be due to excessive scrotal heat. In some situations changing from jockey shorts to boxer shorts may offer a solution. Removal of the heat exposure will usually resolve this type of fertility problem.

It's thought that a *varicocoele* may also damage testicular tissue because of the excessive heat caused by the pooled blood. Some doctors even diagnose varicocoele by measuring the temperature difference between the right and left sides of the scrotum (measuring scrotal temperature, however, is not standardized and is frequently unreliable). If scrotal heat is suspected as a fertility problem, a new device called the testicular hypothermia device (THD) may offer an inexpensive solution. Worn like a jockey strap, the THD cools your testicles to normal levels. Many users report improved semen analysis within a few months. More study is needed before we know who will benefit most from THD use.

If you travel frequently, you may not be able to have sex during your wife's fertile time of the month. For example, due to business commitments, Richard and Margaret B. often found themselves in different cities on her fertile days. With only twelve or thirteen opportunities per year for pregnancy, and with only a 20 percent chance of achieving pregnancy each time, *infrequent sex* can seriously hamper your odds for success. If you have some control over your travel schedule, you can improve your odds for pregnancy by staying at home and having sex during your wife's most fertile days. The rest of the month you can travel all you like. I'll tell you later how to calculate which days are best.

Drugs, Alcohol, and Cigarettes

Since the 1950s more and more people have experimented with *"street" drugs* and many have continued using them, especially marijuana. If you've smoked marijuana over a long period of time, your semen analysis may show lower sperm motility and higher incidences of abnormal sperm morphology. Both of these factors are critical for fertility.

I'd noticed that Richard B. checked marijuana use on his history form, so I wanted to talk with him about it.

I explained, "We don't understand exactly how it works but we do know that there seems to be a correlation between sperm motility and marijuana use. If you want to maximize your chances, I recommend that you stop smoking."

His expression became serious. "Margaret and I have waited a long time for this baby. I'll do anything that will improve our chances."

I don't think Richard was totally convinced, but he did stop smoking. When his semen analysis improved in just two months, I think he was pleasantly surprised.

We also know that central nervous system *depressants* such as barbiturates, heroin, and other narcotics cause impotence and ejaculatory disorders. If you stop using these drugs, usually these symptoms resolve themselves.

Chronic alcohol use can lead to impotence, poor sperm quality, and further complications from liver damage. If alcohol damages your liver, you may have elevated estrogen (female hormone) levels. When a man's female hormones become excessive, they suppress his sex drive and interfere with his sexual performance. If you stop drinking alcohol, these conditions may reverse—provided your liver can recover.

Though not conclusive, there is indication that some of the hundreds of chemicals in *cigarettes* may interfere with fertility by elevating the number of abnormal sperm forms. It's difficult to know, however, how smoking may affect any one individual. If you have concerns about the effects of smoking on you, the best strategy might be to cut down or quit smoking entirely.

Stress and Excessive Exercise

We know that stress and excessive exercise can interrupt the normal flow of hormones from the woman's hypothalamus and pituitary. These abnormal hormone levels can interfere with her menstrual cycles and with her fertility.

Some believe that endorphins (natural narcotics) released by the brain to minimize pain and stress may block the normal release of GnRH, which is essential for maintaining male and female reproductive hormone balance. An example of this would be the abnormal (infrequent or absent) menstrual cycles often seen in women who run fifteen to twenty miles a week. Because of the many similarities in the hypothalamus-pituitary hormone system of men and women, there also may be similarities in their responses to stress and excessive exercise.

If you believe that your life-style is too emotionally or physically stressful, try cutting back. Run fewer miles, try to avoid emotional situations, and incorporate more relaxing activities into your schedule.

Your General Health

Medical Disorders

A number of childhood and adult diseases can adversely affect fertility. Some of the changes are only temporary; for example, a *high fever* (over 102 degrees) may cause your scrotum to overheat and your sperm to die. Usually this type of problem resolves itself in a few months.

Some diseases, however, exert a more lasting effect. For example, *cystic fibrosis, tuberculosis, and adult mumps* can destroy vital testicular tissues and leave you permanently sterile. Consult with your doctor before you write yourself off, however, because these diseases do not affect everyone the same way.

If you have ever contracted *sexually transmitted infections* such as gonorrhea, chlamydia, syphilis, and ureaplasma, scar tissue left by the inflammation can partially or totally block your sperm ducts. Bacteria, viruses, and your own white blood cells (lymphocytes) can attack your sperm and reduce your fertility. Finding white blood cells and dead tissue cells in your semen alerts me to the presence of an active infection. These infections are usually limited to the lower parts of the male genital tract—urethra, prostate, and seminal vesicles. Seldom does the infection travel further in toward your testicles. If infection does reach your testicles, it can cause serious damage.

With the exception of prostatitis, which can be difficult to clear up, sexually transmitted infections will usually respond to antibiotics. If your genitourinary tract becomes scarred from repeated infections, the damaged ducts can often be repaired with microsurgery.

It's vital that your sexual partner also be treated for infection because you can pass the disease back and forth between you. As you'll learn later, sexually transmitted diseases produce far more devastating damage in their female victims.

Systemic diseases such as colitis, diabetes, and hepatitis can deteriorate sperm quality and cause impotence and ejaculatory disorders. When I found that Michael T. had diabetes, for example, I wanted to investigate its effects on his fertility. Sickle-cell anemia, most frequently found in people with black heritage, may also reduce sperm concentration. Insufficient thyroid hormone has also been linked with low sperm motility and other hormone imbalances. I will discuss the specific treatment options available for these disorders in chapter 8.

Kidney problems may also affect your fertility. I remember an executive with a major oil company who developed chronic kidney disease in his mid-forties. He'd had two daughters by his first wife; but his disease-induced fertility problem prevented his new wife from having a child of their own. "My wife really cares desperately about carrying our child," he pleaded. I worked very closely with his nephrologist and together we managed to get him a kidney transplant. With his disease under better control, his sperm count improved, and miraculously the couple produced a baby.

Reports of *breast disorders* such as tenderness, soreness, and milky discharge or *neurological problems* characterized by visual disturbances, dizziness, chronic headaches, and/or seizures may lead me to suspect *multiple sclerosis, nerve damage,* or a problem with the *pituitary*. Since your brain and your master pituitary gland are vital for maintaining your sex hormone balance, any interruption in their function can impair your fertility. I'll discuss the roles your brain and pituitary gland serve in much greater detail in chapter 8.

Surgeries

If you have no sperm in your semen (azospermia), but have normally sized testicles and normal hormone levels, you probably have blockage in the ducts between your testicles and your penis. If a *hernia repair* or *lower abdominal surgery* is part of your medical history, I'd be highly suspicious that you had an accidental vasectomy (severing of the vas deferens or duct coming from the testis during surgery). I remember one man who was quite surprised when I told him that a hernia repair he had when he was six years old caused his fertility problem. After microsurgery to reverse the accidental vasectomy, his sperm count came up to 40 million. Skilled surgeons can reverse both *accidental and elective vasectomies* 90 percent of the time if the reversal is performed within ten years of the vasectomy. Chapter 8 will tell you how this surgery can be done with such precision.

I also need to know if you've incurred nerve damage from a *colon resection*. This injury can cause both erection and ejaculation problems. If you've had *bladder* or *prostate surgery,* you may suffer from retrograde ejaculation. This condition causes you to ejaculate into your bladder instead of out your penis. You can read more about how we manage this problem in chapter 8.

If you've had surgery for the removal of an adrenal, scrotal, or pituitary tumor, I may suspect an endocrine (hormone) imbalance. Once they're correctly diagnosed, hormonal deficiencies often respond well to hormone replacement therapy. The diagnostic procedures and treatment regimens I use for hormonal problems are detailed in the next chapter.

Medications

We know that certain medications lower fertility by depressing sperm production or impairing sexual performance. For example, if you take *high blood pressure medication* (antihypertensives) such as reserpine, methyldopa, and guanethidine; or if you consume alcohol or narcotics, you may have difficulty maintaining an erection and suffer from ejaculation failure. In addition, these drugs can lower your sex drive.

Cytotoxic drugs, anabolic steroids, cimetidine (Tagamet for ulcers), sulfasalazine, spironolactone, opiates, and colchicine all may cause depressed sperm production. We also know that antimalarials, tetracycline, amebicides, nitrofurantoin (for bladder infections), propranolol (Inderal), and barbiturates may cause fertility problems. If you take methotrexate for psoriasis or cancer, you may even suffer irreversible germ cell damage in your testes. Many of the drugs I've mentioned are generic; that is, they are the names for the basic chemical compounds. You can check to see if the medication you're taking contains any of these compounds by looking in the *Physician's Desk Reference* at your library or by asking your doctor. Often by simply altering your medication your doctor can restore your fertility.

Chemotherapy and radiation therapy for cancer may have irreversible effects on fertility. However, if some of your testicular germ cells remain intact, your sperm production may resume when treatment stops. Since every case is individual, you should check with your doctor about your particular situation.

Your Sexual History

Sexual Development

I also need to know about your sexual development. For example, if you had *undescended testes,* I need to know if and when you underwent surgery to correct the problem. If you had the surgery before you were six, your testes may be fine. Otherwise, cellular damage that impairs sperm production may have occurred. It's also helpful for me to know if you went through *puberty* exceptionally early or late (the normal range is nine to sixteen). Sometimes this clues me in to hormone problems.

Sexual Performance

If you have difficulty getting and maintaining an erection, I want to check your general health, your nervous system, your hormone levels, and your exposure to toxic chemicals or medications. Any one of these factors can cause *physical impotence*. If necessary, your doctor may want a second opinion from a psychologist, neurologist, or psychiatrist. I'll discuss more about treating impotence and erection problems in chapter 8.

If you become too excited and almost always ejaculate before inserting your penis into your wife's vagina, you'll never get your sperm into her cervix. And you both will be pretty frustrated with your sexual life. *Premature ejaculation* can often be solved by using the sexual techniques and positions I describe in chapter 8.

I also need to know how often you have sex and what techniques you use. One of my patients told me, for example, that his father had advised him to have sex three times a day. While this "prescription" for pregnancy may sound reasonable, it actually lowered my patient's fertility potential. He could not possibly make enough sperm that frequently.

It's also helpful for me to know if you've previously fathered a child, or if your wife has had an abortion or miscarriage during her partnership with you. With this information I can establish that you were fertile at one time and begin looking for problems that developed since then. *Repeated miscarriages* also alert me to the possibility of a genetic problem with either the man or woman.

Your Family History

Since fertility problems often run in families, I need to know if your mother, father, brothers, or sisters have encountered any difficulties. For example, if your mother had a history of repeated miscarriages when she was pregnant with you, she may have taken a drug called DES. Knowing whether or not you were exposed to DES could help me determine if you're suffering from DES-caused testicular abnormalities. I also need to know if your family has a history of hormonal problems such as diabetes, hypothyroidism, or adrenal gland malfunctions. Adding your family history to other clues may help me decide on which areas to investigate more closely.

Steps for Evaluating Male Fertility

Your doctor will recommend doing a semen analysis and postcoital test. If these are normal, the doctor's focus will shift toward detecting problems with your wife. If your semen analysis reveals abnormalities, however, your doctor will perform a physical examination and various laboratory tests on you. Your doctor will use the results of your abnormal semen analysis and postcoital test (both discussed in chapter 6), to guide the rest of the investigation into your fertility problem. The following discussion will help you understand what procedures and tests are available and when they should be used.

Oligospermia (fewer than 20 million sperm per milliliter)

If your sperm count shows a concentration lower than 20 million sperm per milliliter, I'll first try to eliminate *toxic substances* or recent *illnesses* as possible causes. If your history or life-style does not provide any clues, I will examine your scrotum to determine if your *testicular size* is normal. Underdeveloped testicles may be caused by a number of problems which I discuss in detail later. I will also look for the presence of a *varicocoele* (varicose vein in the scrotum), which may be impairing your sperm production. See chapter 8 for a complete discussion of varicocoeles.

If I find a stress pattern in your semen analysis (low count, poor morphology, and low motility), I'll order blood tests to determine your *hormone levels*. And if I suspect a *genetic problem* such as Klinefelter's syndrome, I may recommend checking your chromosomes (karyotyping). Chapter 8 describes in detail what these tests will reveal and the treatment regimens available for improving sperm production.

If you do not respond to treatment for oligospermia, you are a prime candidate for artificial insemination with your own sperm (AIH) or in vitro fertilization, in which a surgeon retrieves your wife's eggs (ova) and uses your sperm to fertilize them in a petri dish. The fertilized egg (embryo) is then transferred to your wife's uterus in the hope that it will implant and develop into a baby. The first in vitro "miracle baby" was born less than ten years ago. Now in the United States alone over one hundred clinics offer these services. I'll discuss in vitro fertilization and many other technologically advanced options in later chapters.

Severe Oligospermia (fewer than 10 million sperm per milliliter)

If your semen analysis shows fewer than 10 million sperm per milliliter, I will check your *hormone levels* and the *size of your testicles*. I'll measure your *FSH hormone level* to determine if your pituitary gland is stimulating your testes to make sperm. If FSH is elevated (indicating testicular failure) and you are not making sperm, the odds of improving your underlying condition are bleak, although in vitro fertilization may work. If I find that your hormones are deficient and your testicles are small, hormone replacement therapy may help you develop normal testicular function.

When your sperm concentration is this low, I may also recommend that a urologist perform a *testicular biopsy,* which will tell me the condition of your testes at the cellular level. I need to know if your *germ cells* are dividing and producing immature sperm cells. I also want to know if you have *Sertoli, or nurse, cells* to shepherd and nurture the immature sperm cells through their five or so stages of maturation. The biopsy will also tell me if your *Leydig cells* are capable of producing *testosterone* (male hormone), which is vital for sexual performance and sperm development. I can also see if your testicular (seminiferous) tubules are intact. (See figure 8-2 for the male reproductive anatomy.)

If the biopsy reveals that your testicular structures are irreversibly damaged, I probably cannot do anything to improve your sperm production. If the biopsy shows me that your testes are understimulated by hormones, I can prescribe replacement hormones, which may initiate testicular development and establish spermatogenesis. If the biopsy shows me that your testes are normal, then I know that your vas deferens (tube leading from your testicles toward your penis) is partially blocked. Microsurgery may be able to restore the path. Chapter 8 will tell you what can cause these problems and the treatments available to improve oligospermia.

Azospermia

I evaluate azospermia, the condition in which the semen contains no sperm, the same way I evaluate severe oligospermia. However, in addition to performing the tests I do for a severely oligospermic man, I will also test your semen to see if it coagulates and if it contains fructose (sugar). (Azospermic men usually do have semen, because sperm and semen are made in different organs.) Your *seminal vesicles* make fructose and the chemicals that cause your semen to coagulate. If you were born without seminal vesicles or if your ejaculatory duct is blocked, your semen will not coagulate. I may also examine your urine after ejaculation to see if you have retrograde ejaculation. Chapter 8 tells you more about the procedures used to manage these problems.

When Do You Need a Vasogram or Testicular Biopsy?

Vasograms (X rays of your ducts) and biopsies of your testicles may damage delicate genital structures. Therefore, your doctor should exhaust all other measures before using these more invasive diagnostic procedures. With less invasive tests I can predict pretty well whether or not you have an obstruction. However, I must order an *X ray* to determine where an obstruction or absent tubal structure exists. This procedure is usually performed under anesthesia at the same time that you are prepared for corrective surgery.

The following boxes show when a *biopsy* can be helpful and what the biopsy results mean:

When a Testicular Biopsy Can Be Helpful

1. If you have severe oligospermia or azospermia; low or normal FSH levels; and do not respond to hormone replacement therapy.

2. If you are azospermic; have normal hormone levels and normal testicular size.

Interpreting Testicular Biopsy Findings

1. If you are azospermic and have a normal testes biopsy, you definitely have a *tubal blockage*. (See chapter 8 for a complete discussion of tubal blockage and corrective techniques.)

2. If you are oligospermic because your testes are performing at an abnormally slow rate, you have *hypospermatogenesis*.

3. If you are azospermic because your testes cannot complete the sperm maturation process, you have *maturation arrest*.

Hypospermatogenesis

If the biopsy finds hypospermatogenesis (perhaps a phase of maturation arrest), you will show diminished germ (germination) cell activity and marked germ cell loss. Since the germ cells are the precursors of sperm, you will produce low numbers of sperm or no sperm at all. Chemical toxins, drugs, and varicocoeles may cause hypospermatogenesis.

Maturation Arrest

With maturation arrest, one of the most frequent biopsy findings in male fertility, your germ cells divide and produce early sperm forms, and other testicular structures will appear normal. At one stage in their maturation, however, *sperm development halts throughout all your testicular tubules*. The condition may be complete (azospermic) or partial (oligospermic). Chemical toxins, drugs, and varicocoeles may cause maturation arrest. If your FSH level is high, indicating severe testicular damage, it may be too late for treatment. However, things are brighter if your FSH level is low or normal. Removing the toxins and/or repairing your varicocoele will often restore spermatogenesis.

8. Maximizing
Male Fertility Potential

"Dr. Perloe, we keep getting conflicting information about male fertility treatment. Could you clarify the current thinking for us?" the RESOLVE leader asked.

"The first part of the male formula is what I call *pretesticular function*. This means that your hormone system must be functioning properly in order to stimulate your testicles to make sperm.

"The second ingredient I call the *testicular component*. This means that when stimulated by your sex hormones, your testicles must be capable of producing sperm. Testicles can be congenitally deformed or they can be damaged by chemical toxins, illness, systemic disease, or trauma." I saw Steven S.'s hand go up. "Yes, Steven?"

"But I thought your testicles *made* your sex hormones. If your testicles aren't working, how can your hormones be stimulating them?"

"Your testicles do produce the male hormone testosterone. However, your brain and your pituitary gland, located at the base of your brain, produce chemicals that tell your testicles *when* to make testosterone and *when* to make sperm. Without these signals from your brain and pituitary, your testicles may fail to mature and fail to make sperm.

"The third ingredient of the male fertility formula is *posttesticular function*. The ducts leading from your sperm-producing testicles must provide a clear and continuous path for your sperm to travel out of your penis. Congenital tubal defects, surgeries, and blockage from infections may clog up these pathways."

"What can be done for blocked tubes?" Michael T. asked.

"Today with the aid of microsurgery, most tubal problems can be corrected, including vasectomy reversals."

I turned to the chalkboard and wrote down the fourth factor, *ejaculatory disturbances, impotence, and sexual problems*. "These are the final ingredients of the male fertility formula," I said. "You must be able to deliver your sperm to your wife's cervix in order to make a baby." I set the chalk in the tray and turned back toward the group.

"There are some exceptions to this. Some delivery problems can be overcome with artificial insemination. For example, some men ejaculate backward into the bladder. When this happens, we can retrieve the ejaculated sperm and use artificial insemination techniques to get the sperm to their destination."

"What if the man can't perform?" a woman across the room asked.

"There are two types of sexual performance problems—physiological impotence and psychological impotence. Often it's difficult to separate the two, since men with impaired sexual performance frequently have psychological problems regardless of the source of their difficulty. Physiological impotence may be caused by toxic chemicals, hormone deficiencies, "street" drugs, medications, and nerve damage, for example. A complete fertility evaluation should reveal the source of the problem. And even with physiological impotence, counseling may be needed to ease the difficulties associated with inadequate sexual performance.

"These are the four ingredients necessary for male fertility." I started toward my chair. "If any one of them is out of order, you may have a fertility problem. Working together, you and your physician must identify the deficient factor and direct treatment toward improving that function."

Male Fertility: How It Works

The Male Hormone System

The Hypothalamus and Pituitary Start the Action

Approximately every ninety minutes a specialized area in your brain (hypothalamus) secretes GnRH (gonadotropic-releasing hormone). GnRH signals your pituitary gland, located at the base of your brain, to produce LH (luteinizing hormone) and FSH (follicle-stimulating hormone). (See figure 8-1.)

LH tells your testes to secrete the male hormone *testosterone*. Testosterone stimulates your sexual desires and develops and maintains your male secondary sex characteristics such as hair growth and deep voice. Together, testosterone and FSH stimulate your testes to produce sperm (spermatogenesis). Your body's ability to make and regulate these hormones is vital for maintaining your virility and sperm production.

Feedback Hormones from Your Testicles

You have feedback hormones—testosterone and inhibin—that keep a check and balance on your GnRH, LH, and FSH levels. Once the Leydig cells in your testicles produce enough testosterone, your hormone control systems cut back on GnRH and LH production. When the Sertoli cells, which

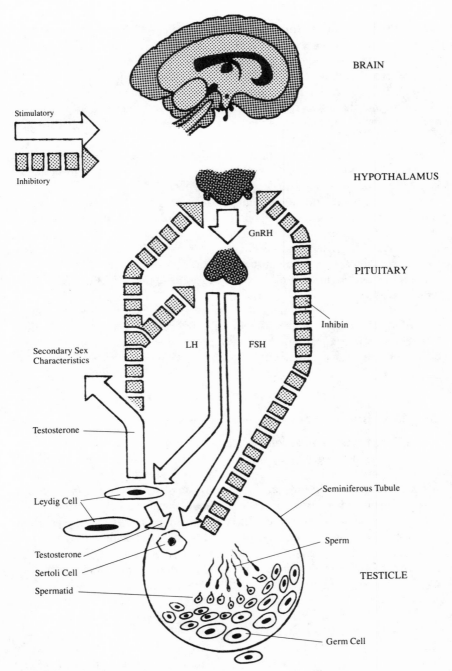

Figure 8-1. Male Hormone System

respond to FSH stimulation, produce enough inhibin, the pituitary cuts back FSH production. Examining figure 8-1 will help you visualize your fertility hormone control system. These relationships will become more clear in the discussions that follow.

The Stages of Sperm Production

Cell Division

Each day your testicles make millions of sperm. (See figure 8–2.) Your testicles are composed of a number of different types of cells which support and surround masses of microscopic seminiferous tubules. Your sperm grow and mature within these tubules. The germ cells (germinal cells or basic sperm cell factories) line these tubule walls. When they are stimulated by the Sertoli cells, the germ cells divide (mitosis) to produce one primary spermatocyte that contains a full complement of your forty-six chromosomes (genetic material). The germ cells remain intact to divide repeatedly throughout your reproductive life. The primary spermatocytes, containing forty-six chromosomes, however, proceed to divide by a special process called meiosis. Meiosis produces four spermatids (immature sperm) containing twenty-three chromosomes each. These spermatids are destined to fertilize your wife's egg, containing twenty-three of her chromosomes. At this point cell division ends and the sperm maturation process begins.

Sperm Maturation

The spermatids remain attached to your tubule wall, where they are nurtured by the Sertoli, or nurse, cells. It takes about ninety days for the sperm to grow, mature, and travel through the tubules to a central storage area called the epididymis. Here the sperm become powerful swimmers. After each ejaculation, it takes about forty hours for your epididymis to refill with mature sperm (this is why too-frequent intercourse can impair fertility).

Each microscopic sperm carries all the genetic information necessary to fertilize the egg. Half of your sperm carry an X chromosome (inherited from your mother) and half carry a Y chromosome (inherited from your father). If an X-carrying sperm fertilizes your wife's egg (ovum), you'll have a baby girl. If a Y-carrying sperm fertilizes the ovum, you'll have a baby boy. In this way the husband's genetic contribution determines the baby's sex.

The Sperm Delivery System

When you ejaculate, your sperm rush through a number of channels between your epididymis and the opening of your penis. (You can view the course that your sperm travel during ejaculation in figure 8-2.) At the moment of ejaculation, your epididymis expels the sperm into the pulsating muscular walls of your vas deferens. While coursing through your vas deferens, the sperm pass the seminal vesicles. These secrete fructose (a sugar to feed your

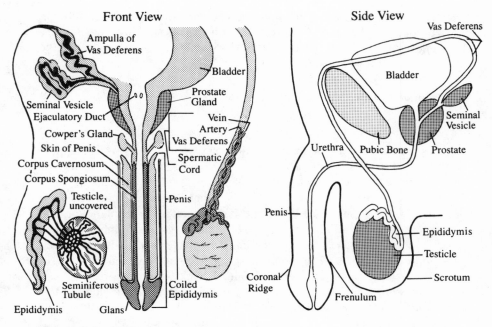

Figure 8-2. Male Anatomy

sperm), seminal fluids (to protect your sperm), and a chemical that coagulates your semen soon after it enters your wife's vagina. Then your sperm speed through your ejaculatory ducts past your prostate gland, which secretes additional seminal fluids, including a chemical that liquefies your coagulated semen within an hour after ejaculation. As your semen (sperm plus your seminal fluids) rushes past the bladder, a muscle (sphincter) squeezes the bladder opening shut. This guides the semen on course through your urethra and out of your penis.

Erection, Orgasm, and Ejaculation

Erection, orgasm, and ejaculation are three distinct processes controlled both by your conscious mind and by involuntary neural responses. To get sperm to your wife's cervix, all three of these processes must be working properly.

Erection
Erection may occur when you have an erotic thought or when your penis is touched. During an erection, nerves signal the blood vessels in your erectile tissue to dilate and become engorged, and your penis swells and becomes rigid. Friction from manual and vaginal stimulation sends more signals to the

brain and stimulates orgasm and ejaculation. Psychological factors can stimulate or interfere with your erection; however, once you reach orgasm your automatic reflex actions run their course.

Orgasm and Ejaculation

Orgasm is the name given to the physiological and sensory thrill that accompanies ejaculation. The first stage of orgasm, called *ejaculatory inevitability,* occurs two to four seconds before ejaculation. During this interval you sense your imminent ejaculation and cannot continue to control the process. Your prostate gland and your seminal vesicles start to pulse. The second stage of orgasm begins when you involuntarily expel semen in several convulsive waves. Typically you ejaculate about one teaspoon of semen, which contains 40 to 150 million sperm. The first squirt (semen fraction) generally contains the largest number of sperm.

After orgasm, most men and many women experience a *recovery (refractory) period* during which they cannot have another orgasm. This period may last many minutes and sometimes several hours. You may also experience an erection refractory period.

As I discuss the various causes of male fertility problems, the statistics in table 8-1 will help you place each condition into proper perspective.

Table 8-1
The Most Common Male Fertility Problems

Problem	% Infertile Population
Hormone	
Endocrine	9
Hyperprolactinemia (elevated prolactin)	10–40
Congenital adrenal hyperplasia	1
Stress	?
Sperm Production	
Varicocoele	40
Testicular failure	14
Smoking, heat, drugs	?
Sperm Delivery	
Obstructed ducts	7
Congenital obstruction/absence of ducts	2
Erection, Orgasm, Ejaculation	
Sexual problems	5
Ejaculation problems	2

The Male Fertility Formula:
Where Can Things Go Wrong?

In the rest of this chapter I will describe how each of the four fertility factors may malfunction, how specific disorders can be diagnosed, and how they can be corrected.

Fertility Factor #1: The Hormone Balancing Act

Several things can go wrong with your hypothalamus-pituitary endocrine system:

- Your brain can fail to pulse GnRH properly.
- Your pituitary can fail to produce enough LH and FSH to stimulate your testes.
- Your testes' Leydig cells may not produce testosterone in response to LH (pituitary) stimulation.
- Your body may produce other hormones and chemical compounds which interfere with your sex-hormone balance.

Any one of these conditions can impair your sperm production. To help you understand the treatment for these hormonal disorders, I'd like to explain what medications are available and how they are prescribed to improve male fertility.

An Overview of Hormonal Treatment

If your pituitary hormones (LH and FSH) are low, but you do have a working hypothalamus and pituitary gland, clomiphene citrate (Serophene, Clomid) should stimulate your hypothalamus to pulse GnRH at regular intervals. When your hypothalamus properly releases GnRH, your pituitary gland will respond by producing LH and FSH. If Serophene does *not* improve LH and FSH levels, then I will suspect that your pituitary gland may be malfunctioning. (Since Serophene is an oral medication, it is more convenient and less expensive than your other options.)

If your pituitary cannot manufacture the missing sex hormones, you can take hormone supplements. Injections of hCG (human chorionic gonadotropin) will increase your LH supply and often stimulate your testes to produce testosterone and sperm. If your response to hCG is inadequate, I might add Pergonal (FSH and LH) to stimulate sperm production. Pergonal and hCG treatments can be quite expensive, since they require regularly repeated injections.

If these treatment regimens are successful, sperm production and quality will begin to improve within three to four months.

Diagnosing and Treating Specific Hormonal Problems

Hyperprolactinemia

Hyperprolactinemia (elevated prolactin) can be difficult to diagnose because your FSH, LH, and testosterone levels will be normal. We find elevated prolactin, a hormone associated with nursing mothers, in 10 to 40 percent of infertile males. Mild prolactin elevation produces no symptoms; however, greater elevations can reduce sperm production, impair your sex drive, and cause impotence. Hyperprolactinemia responds well to a drug called Parlodel (bromocriptine). A prolactin-secreting tumor will also respond to Parlodel; however, surgery and/or radiation therapy may be necessary.

Hypothyroidism

Found in 1 percent of infertile men, hypothyroidism (low thyroid hormone) can cause poor semen quality, poor testicular function, and/or disturbances in sex drive. You will be lethargic, intolerant of cold, and overweight. Because the pituitary gland is trying its best to stimulate your unresponsive thyroid gland, your pituitary-produced TSH (thyroid-stimulating hormone) level will be elevated. Elevated prolactin levels, frequently found with this disorder, may cause impotence.

You can sometimes bring on hypothyroidism by eating a diet high in iodine—for example, kelp or seaweed—or taking multimineral tablets. Chronic ingestion of iodides in cough syrups (formerly used in treating asthmatic bronchitis) may also produce these symptoms. In addition, hypothyroidism may be caused by radioactive thyroid medications and autoimmune diseases.

Correcting your diet or beginning thyroid hormone replacement therapy should elevate your sperm count to previous levels. I must emphasize that unless you have low thyroid, thyroid hormone replacement therapy will not improve your sperm quality.

Stress and Excessive Exercise

When a woman is under a great deal of stress, we can use Serophene to regulate the GnRH pulses from her hypothalamus and restore ovulation. It seems logical to assume that Serophene may help a man in the same situation. Although we don't know the therapeutic effects for certain, I have observed some semen improvement when Serophene has been used with these men.

I especially remember Ted M., who was the typical "Type A" personality. Ted had a borderline sperm count, smoked five packs of cigarettes and drank ten cups of coffee a day, and was a workaholic. I prescribed Serophene and also counseled with him about restructuring his habits. With some help from his friends in RESOLVE, Ted began a moderate exercise program and got his nicotine and caffeine habits under control. Within five months his count began improving and a year later he fathered a child.

Congenital Adrenal Hyperplasia

Found in 1 percent of infertile males, congenital adrenal hyperplasia may be suspected when a semen analysis shows a low sperm count, an increased number of immature sperm cells, sperm with long tapered heads, and low motility. These abnormalities occur when the pituitary is suppressed by increased levels of adrenal androgens. Men with this disease may also have hypertension (high blood pressure) and edema (water retention). Early onset of the disease may result in ambiguous genitalia at birth or reaching puberty at an early age. Adult onset may be characterized by infertility, high blood pressure, and/or water retention.

Cortisone replacement therapy will lower your androgens and allow your pituitary to function normally. Therefore, indirectly, cortisone replacement therapy will elevate your sperm count.

Some of these situations are not so easily managed. One time I had the unfortunate job of counseling one of my bearded male patients who was genetically a *she*. Because the adrenal androgens (male hormones) had dominated this person's hormonal system since before birth, male secondary sex characteristics developed. Fortunately this finding is quite rare.

Hypogonadotropic Hypopituitarism

Hypogonadotropic hypopituitarism is a spectrum of diseases with a complicated name that means low *(hypo-)* pituitary gland output of LH and FSH. Other stages of this disease are called *isolated gonadotropin defect* and *panhypopituitarism*, in which the entire *(pan-)* pituitary gland is affected.

These diseases arrest sperm development and cause the progressive loss of germ cells from the testes. In addition, the seminiferous tubules and Leydig cells (which produce testosterone) also deteriorate. If the condition persists for a long time, you will have no sperm production at all. (See chapter 7 for a discussion of maturation arrest.) When the disease is associated with a pituitary tumor, elevated prolactin levels may also cause impotence.

Clifford J. showed signs typical of this progressive degeneration. Over a period of three to four years he gradually lost his heavy beard, became less interested in sex, and eventually could not sustain an erection. His blood tests revealed low LH, FSH, and testosterone levels, and his sperm count was 10 million per milliliter. I prescribed Serophene in hopes of improving his sperm count and sexual performance. Fortunately he responded to the drug, and six months later his sperm count increased to 18 million. After performing AIH four times, his wife became pregnant. Following fertility treatment, I discontinued the Serophene (it's too expensive to take all of the time) and continued giving him a testosterone supplement to maintain his virility and sexual performance.

Panhypopituitarism

Complete pituitary gland failure (panhypopituitarism) lowers your growth hormone, ACTH level, thyroid-stimulating hormone (TSH), and LH and FSH levels. If you have this rare disease, you will have multiple symptoms that include impotence, decreased sex drive, loss of secondary sex characteristics, and normal or undersized testicles. Your hypothyroidism (low thyroid hormone) will cause you to gain weight, be intolerant of cold, and feel lethargic. If the disorder began early enough in your life, you may even be a dwarf. The hormonal deficiency is often caused by a tumor, surgery, or trauma to the pituitary gland.

No amount of stimulation can improve the performance of the damaged pituitary gland, so I will work with an endocrinologist to supplement the missing pituitary hormones. The thyroid hormone supplement as well as other hormone replacements will restore general health and vigor. At that point I administer hCG to stimulate the testicles to produce testosterone and to begin making sperm.

Kallman's Syndrome

Kallman's syndrome is a congenital hypothalamic dysfunction. If you are born with this unusual condition, you will have underdeveloped testicles and possibly a harelip, cleft palate, color blindness, and/or the inability to smell. Affected men have varying degrees of sexual infantilism (prepuberty) and no sperm production. Since the hypothalamus fails to stimulate the pituitary adequately, FSH, LH, and testosterone levels are low. I treat Kallman's syndrome similarly to hypogonadotropic hypopituitarism. Although at first it seems hopeless, men afflicted with Kallman's syndrome can achieve normal puberty and eventually become fertile.

Delayed Puberty

Individuals with isolated pituitary growth hormone deficiency do not sexually mature until their mid to late twenties. Hormone supplements can make them look virile, but until they go through puberty, they won't be fertile. Pergonal and/or hCG injections can bring on puberty, although if left alone, sexual maturity and fertility will be achieved in time.

Fertile Eunuch

If you have this rare disorder, your virilization (acquisition of adult sex characteristics) will be moderately advanced, but you will not have completed sexual maturation and testicular growth. If I biopsied your rather small testicles (a procedure not usually needed to diagnose this condition), I'd find evidence of sperm production and thus the potential for fertility. Since the arrest of sperm production and low testosterone levels are caused by an LH deficiency, administering hCG will raise both hormone levels and stimulate sperm production.

Fertility Factor #2: Treating Unresponsive Testicles

What Causes Testicular Failure?

Let's suppose that your hypothalamus and pituitary are working well. The fact is that some conditions prevent your testicles from *responding* to pituitary hormone stimulation. Testicular failure, as it's called, can be caused by genetic abnormalities or by damage from drugs, injury, radiation, excess heat, adult mumps, a varicocoele, or toxins from your environment. Sensing abnormal testicular function, your brain responds by telling your pituitary to pump out more FSH to stimulate sperm production. In fact, elevated FSH is the primary diagnostic indicator for testicular failure.

Unfortunately there isn't much that can be done for *primary testicular failure,* which is caused by a genetic mistake. The malformed testes are unable to produce sperm and no amount of stimulation will improve their function. However, if you have this problem, you and your wife need not go childless. You are a prime candidate for artificial insemination with donor sperm (AID). With AID your baby will inherit your wife's genes and traits and will be your own through your marital bonds and love. I'll talk more about AID techniques in a later chapter.

We have a better chance of treating *secondary testicular failure* (acquired damage). If, before too much testicular damage occurs, you discontinue potentially harmful medications and illicit drugs; avoid contact with toxic substances such as pesticides; reduce excess heat exposure; or have a varicocoele surgically repaired, you may once again produce sperm. Below is a discussion of what causes testicular failure and the methods available for improving fertility.

Varicocoele

When I examined Steven S., I could see his varicocoele as I crossed the room:

"Steven, see these veins crisscrossing over the left side of your scrotum?"

He leaned over for a better view. "Oh, those. I've had those for years. They never give me any trouble."

"They're called a varicocoele—a varicose vein that allows blood to pool in your scrotum. It's thought that poor circulation may lead to a buildup of blood toxins or increase your scrotal temperature. Either of these conditions may result in what's called a *testicular stress pattern.*

"The typical stress pattern shows depressed sperm production, poor sperm motility, and poor sperm morphology—which is exactly what your semen analysis showed. I also noticed that your left testicle is a bit small. That's another frequent finding with varicocoeles."

"Is that why I'm infertile?"

"It could be," I answered. "Forty percent of infertile men have varicocoeles."

"What can you do about it?"

"With some men I'd try artificial insemination with their sperm. If that didn't work, I'd get a second opinion from a urologic surgeon. There is some evidence that repairing the vein may improve your chances of having a baby to at least fifty-fifty. However, with your 15 million count and 20 percent motility, it's my guess your chances for AIH working aren't very good.

"I'd like you to see a urologic surgeon. You should know, however, that 10 percent of normally fertile men have varicocoeles. So there are no guarantees that the varicocoele is causing your marginal count or that repairing it will improve your fertility."

A *varicocoele* is a dilation of the veins that carry blood out of your scrotum. The bulging veins cannot support the column of blood returning to your circulatory system, so your blood pools in the swollen vessels surrounding your testicles. Because of the venous structure, varicocoeles usually occur on your left side. How they cause infertility is unknown, but it is speculated that poor circulation (toxic buildup) and/or higher scrotal heat from pooling blood may be factors.

Two-thirds of the infertile men who have a varicocoele also have reduced sperm motility and abnormal sperm morphology. The semen will contain large numbers of sperm with tapered heads and many immature spermatids. If these findings are coupled with smaller than normal testicular size, you probably have a varicocoele.

A pronounced varicocoele feels like a "bag of worms" in the scrotum. Your doctor may find a less obvious varicocoele by having you bend over and exert a downward pressure as though you are forcing a bowel movement. The pressure will force the veins to bulge out. Other tests used to diagnose varicocoele include the Doppler stethoscope (ultrasound) and thermography (thermal detection methods). If the temperature difference between one side of your scrotum and the other is significant, you probably have a varicocoele. Unfortunately the instruments and techniques used to measure this small temperature difference have not been perfected. These diagnostic procedures are not painful and are relatively inexpensive.

Varicocoele Treatment

Corrective surgery is not always necessary because laboratory techniques for improving semen quality may provide an adequate sample for intrauterine insemination. For example, your semen can be collected, concentrated, and washed for artificial insemination (AIH).

Varicocoele repair is one of the primary methods used to improve sperm motility and concentration. Surgical correction of the varicocoele will improve semen quality in 70 percent of infertile men, and 50 percent of their wives become pregnant. When the surgery works, as it did for Steven, improved sperm motility seems to be the most significant result. If you rate varicocoele surgery by improvement in semen quality, Steven's results were nominal. His count improved to 20 million and his motility to 40 percent. However, if you ask Steven and Kathy to rate his improvement by the final results—a delightful baby girl—they would say the surgery was 100 percent successful.

Currently research is being done to determine which people will benefit most from varicocoele surgery. I feel that the sperm penetration assay (SPA) and acrosin test (see description below) show the most promise. Sometimes called the hamster penetration test, the SPA predicts the ability of your sperm to penetrate an egg for fertilization. By mixing your sperm with specially prepared hamster eggs, we can see if your sperm can penetrate the hamster egg membrane. If your sperm penetrate these eggs, your sperm should be able to penetrate your wife's egg. Unfortunately the SPA costs between $300 and $400 to perform, so it is not ordered as routinely as the semen analysis.

Research seems to indicate that if you have a relatively normal semen analysis and a positive sperm penetration assay (your sperm penetrated the hamster ova) or acrosin test, varicocoele surgery may not be appropriate. In other words, *if your sperm are functional, varicocoele repair probably won't improve your fertility potential.* AIH may be more appropriate.

If your SPA is negative (your sperm cannot penetrate the hamster ova), varicocoele repair may improve your sperm quality. If, however, your SPA remains negative after varicocoele surgery, pregnancy is unlikely.

The acrosin test (costing only twenty dollars) may not only replace the SPA but may provide additional information. By directly measuring sperm enzymes, this test predicts the sperm's ability to penetrate the protein outer layer of the egg (zona pellucida) *and* the egg membrane. It's possible that soon the semen analysis together with the acrosin test will be used to screen candidates for varicocoele surgery. I'll discuss the significance of this test more thoroughly in chapter 18.

Undescended Testicles (Cryptorchidism)

Undescended testicles occur in 8 out of 1,000 boys. Since some testicles descend during the first year, making a diagnosis before one year of age is difficult. If only one testicle is affected, fertility will not be compromised. However, there's a 20 percent increased incidence of cancer in the normal testicle. (Normal risk for testicular cancer is 8 in 100,000 men.)

If the undescended testicles are surgically lowered before age six, normal fertility will be preserved. If the repair is done after age six, however, irreversible damage to the seminiferous tubules will cause infertility. These men will appear virile, but they have a forty to fifty times greater risk of developing testicular cancer.

Infection

Mumps, tuberculosis, brucellosis, gonorrhea, typhoid, influenza, smallpox, and syphilis can cause your testes to atrophy. With some of these infections your LH and testosterone (virility) levels may remain normal. However, if your FSH is high, as in Pete B.'s case, the prognosis for testicular recovery is poor.

When he was seventeen, Pete B., the son of one of my patients, caught the mumps from his little brother. Both testes were affected, one side more than the other. When I saw him in his early twenties, Pete had scanty pubic hair and complained about having no sex drive. His semen analysis showed a sperm count of 10 million, with 30 percent motility, and his FSH was elevated. Together this evidence told me that Pete had suffered extensive testicular damage.

To relieve his immediate concerns about his manliness I prescribed testosterone replacement to restore his virility. Bolstered by his newfound sexual abilities, he married and soon returned for fertility counseling. Since Pete's count was so low I suggested they first try AIH. "If AIH doesn't work within four or five cycles, in vitro fertilization will give you a good chance for a baby." I have to give them credit. They stuck with the AIH regimen for five tries. It was worth it: Pete has a cute red-haired, green-eyed baby girl who's got him wrapped around her little finger. And Grandmother shows me her pictures every time she comes in for an appointment.

Torsion

Torsion of the testis and/or blood vessels supplying the testis (spermatic cord) is a common problem that threatens fertility. Torsion is caused by a supportive tissue abnormality which allows the testis to twist inside your scrotum, causing extreme pain and swelling. When your gonad rotates, the attached blood vessels entwine like the ropes on a swing and pinch shut the blood supply. Within a few hours cellular degeneration from impaired blood flow begins to take its toll. The amount of cellular damage varies with the degree of torsion; however, emergency surgery must be performed to prevent further damage.

Due to rapid growth of the body during puberty, torsion seems to occur most frequently at that age. If you have torsion on one side, you have a 40 percent chance of having torsion on the other side, too. Consequently the surgeon should secure the unaffected testis to prevent subsequent trauma.

When the deteriorated testis is left in place, damage is often induced in the unaffected testis. Studies suggest that removing the damaged testis may help preserve full function and fertility of the remaining one.

Trauma

Severe injury to your testicles requires prompt intervention to avoid tissue loss. If you have marked swelling and pain, a surgeon should explore your scrotum and make needed repairs. When required, a surgeon can drain a clot of blood from the scrotum (scrotal hemotoma) or repair a testicular rupture.

Klinefelter's Syndrome

Each cell in a normal man's body has only one Y (male) and one X (female) chromosome. People with Klinefelter's syndrome, however, have one Y and two X chromosomes in each cell. On examination I will find peanut-sized testes and enlarged breasts. A chromosome analysis (karyotyping) will confirm this diagnosis.

In the beginning stages of this rare disorder your FSH is only slightly elevated, indicating minimal testicular failure. Administration of hCG at this stage may improve sperm production. However, eventually all of the active testicular structures will atrophy, including germ cells, tubules, Leydig cells, and Sertoli cells; the testes themselves actually shrink. After testicular failure occurs (causing FSH levels to rise dramatically), improving fertility is impossible. However, these people can still have children by using artificial insemination with donor sperm.

Cushing's Syndrome

Cushing's syndrome occurs when the adrenal gland secretes excessive amounts of cortisol. People with this rare disorder will have a moon-shaped face and will suffer from water retention, obesity, impotence, feminized characteristics, loss of sex drive, and infertility. The condition may be due to an adrenal tumor or to excessive stimulation of the adrenal gland by ACTH (adrenocorticotropic hormone) from the pituitary. If ACTH is high, either the pituitary is overactive or an ACTH-secreting pituitary tumor is present (called *Cushing's disease*).

Elevated adrenal androgens suppress LH and FSH production and spermatogenesis. Cortisone replacement therapy will reduce cortisol levels and restore natural LH, FSH, and sperm production. If a tumor is present, surgery and/or radiation therapy is required.

Germ Cell Aplasia (Sertoli Cell Only)

Germ cell aplasia (Sertoli cell only) is an inherited condition. The testicular biopsy will show that the slightly small testes have normal Leydig cells, no germ cells, and narrow tubules. Because their Leydig cells continue to produce testosterone, these men remain virile, but they cannot produce sperm.

Germ cell aplasia can also be caused by exposure to large doses of radiation and prolonged exposure to toxic substances. Once the damage is complete, no therapy is available. To couples facing this diagnosis, I usually suggest artificial insemination with donor sperm or adoption.

Testicular Enzyme Defects

Testicular enzyme defects prevent the testes from responding normally to hormonal stimulation. These rare genetic defects can cause multiple genital abnormalities, incomplete virilization, small testes, and low or no sperm production. LH and FSH will both be high, since the brain is doing its best to stimulate the unresponsive testicles. Providing some sperm production still exists, AIH or in vitro fertilization may lead to pregnancy.

Fertility Factor #3: Repairing Sperm Ducts

Seven percent of infertile men cannot transport sperm from their testicles out of their penis. The path from each of your testicles to your penis may be interrupted by a number of conditions:

- A genetic or developmental mistake may cause blockage and/or the absence of one or both tubes (vasa).
- Scarring from tuberculosis or sexually transmitted diseases such as gonorrhea and chlamydia may block your epididymis or tubes.
- An elective or accidental vasectomy (severing of the vasa) may interrupt tube continuity.

I usually suspect an obstruction when you have normal-sized testes and normal hormone levels but fewer than 1 million sperm per milliliter of ejaculate. If you have a *partial obstruction,* your sperm count and motility will be low and you will have an increased percentage of abnormal sperm morphology. *Complete obstruction* results in the total absence of sperm and, depending on the location of the obstruction, possibly the absence of semen. Twenty-five percent of azospermic men have duct obstructions. Unfortunately, if you're missing large sections of the vas, surgical repair is impossible. (See "The Artificial Spermatocoele" below.)

If I suspect an obstruction, I will order an X ray of your tubes to locate the exact position of the obstruction or missing section. Surgical repair is usually performed at the same time as the X ray, since both require general anesthesia. I'd like to describe each type of transport problem and tell you how they are diagnosed and corrected.

Voluntary or Accidental Vasectomy

Voluntary vasectomy (surgical dissection of both vasa deferentia for birth control) is the most common posttesticular cause of fertility loss. A vasectomy may also occur accidentally as a complication of traumatic injury, scrotal surgery, and lower abdominal surgery such as a hernia repair.

Infection and Disease

Chronic active prostatitis and gonococcal or tuberculosis *infections* can cause scarring and tubal blockage. I suspect these diseases if you have difficulty voiding, show a urethral discharge, or have a painful and enlarged prostate gland on rectal examination. The tail of the epididymis at its junction with the vas deferens is the usual site of this type of obstruction. The seminal vesicles, prostate, and ejaculatory ducts may also be involved.

Azospermic men with acquired obstruction usually have fructose in their seminal fluid and normal FSH levels, indicating that the seminal vesicles and testes are intact and functional. If I have any doubts about my diagnosis, I'll order a testicular biopsy to confirm normal sperm production.

Performing microsurgery to repair the epididymis is tedious, but the 50 to 70 percent success rate approaches that of vasectomy reversals.

Cystic fibrosis, an inherited disease occurring in 1 out of 2,500 live births, may also cause low sperm counts, diminished semen volume, or the congenital absence of the vas deferens.

Congenital Obstruction

Congenital abnormalities account for approximately 2 percent of male fertility problems. Frequently the blockage will be located at the anatomical junction between your vas and your epididymis. If fructose is absent from your seminal fluid, I suspect congenital absence of both the vasa and seminal vesicles or a rare obstruction of the ejaculatory ducts. Congenital malformations are frequently difficult to overcome, since many times long sections of both vasa may be absent.

I remember one unusual situation involving a couple in their mid-twenties. Jess H.'s semen analysis showed no sperm at all. On his history form he indicated that his mother had taken DES to prevent miscarriage. Because I suspected blockage from the usage of this drug while he was in utero, I referred him to a urologic microsurgeon for X rays and a biopsy. In the meantime I completed a fertility workup on his wife and confirmed that she was fertile. (It wouldn't make much sense for them to pay for expensive microsurgery on him if she had a serious fertility problem.) Jess's X ray showed blockage at the epididymis on both sides, so the surgeon repaired the tubes. After several months Jess's semen analysis showed marked improvement.

Vasectomy Reversal and Surgical Repair for Obstruction

Today more and more men want vasectomy reversals. Often they find themselves divorcing and remarrying in midlife and then wanting to begin a new family. Fortunately, if your reversal is performed within ten years of the original vasectomy, you have a 70 to 90 percent chance of restoring your fertility.

After ten years the prolonged pressure buildup from sperm in your epididymis may "blow out" holes in the epididymis wall. These ruptures can be difficult to correct. In addition, you may begin to form antibodies against your own sperm. Later I'll discuss the adverse affects of sperm antibodies in greater detail.

Vasectomy reversal and tubal repairs are complicated by the fact that the vas has a thick, tough muscular wall with a pencil-lead-sized opening (lumen) inside the tube. Pressure from sperm production tends to swell or enlarge the portion of the tube attached to the epididymis. Thus the lumen will be larger in diameter than the detached tube leading to the penis. Fitting the two ends together can be tedious, but gentle dilation of the smaller tube and microsurgical techniques seem to work well.

The Artificial Spermatocoele

When your vas deferens are scarred and blocked over a long segment or if they are absent altogether, surgical reconnection is not possible. In these situations a few surgeons have tried creating an artificial spermatocoele, or pouch, into which the sperm can collect. The doctor can then retrieve the sperm for artificial insemination. One study resulted in the recovery of sperm from 33 percent of the men and pregnancy in 10 percent of their wives. In my experience the results have been very poor because the collected sperm are not mature enough to swim and fertilize the egg. At this time I cannot recommend the procedure. Perhaps in the near future a silicone prosthesis will be perfected and approved for this use.

One research project in Australia has started two pregnancies from sperm retrieved directly from the epididymis. Further studies may provide new hope for these couples.

Fertility Factor #4: How We Correct Ejaculatory Disturbances

Impotence

You are impotent if you are unable to maintain an erection and ejaculate during sex. *Organic impotence* differs from *psychological impotence* in that with organic impotence your body cannot respond because of insufficient hormone stimulation, incomplete nerve paths, and/or insufficient reproductive organ development. Some people have always been impotent *(primary impotence)* and others may develop impotence later in life as a result of surgery, injury, or an illness. Determining the cause of impotence is not as straightforward as one would like because many men who suffer from organic impotence may also have a number of psychological problems stemming from their inability to perform sexually.

Impotence can be caused by diseases such as prostatitis, diabetes, and kidney failure and by neurological disorders such as multiple sclerosis and spinal injuries. Impotence may also be caused by pelvic surgery, including kidney transplant, prostate, and bladder surgery. Hormone imbalances such as elevated prolactin and low testosterone levels can also decrease sex drive and cause impotence. Many drugs and medications such as antihypertensives, alcohol, and narcotics have been linked with impotence.

Men with organic impotence have few if any erections during their sleep. You can confirm if you have organic impotence by monitoring your nocturnal erections for several nights. You can do this with an expensive overnight hospital testing procedure. Or you can do it at home more simply with my "trading stamp procedure." Just before going to bed moisten a short strip of trading stamps and stick them in a circle around the center of your penis. Make sure the ends of the strip overlap and the stamps glue together securely. If the strip breaks during the night, you probably had a nocturnal erection. Repeat the procedure several nights in a row to make sure.

If your impotence is due to a hormone imbalance and/or systemic disease, appropriate treatment may alleviate your problem. Or supplementing your testosterone to normal levels may improve your sexual desires and performance.

You can overcome irreversible organic impotence with a surgical *penile implant*. Thousands of men use them, and many of their wives report that during intercourse they cannot sense any difference from a normal erection. Nearly half of the penile implants have been used with men having diabetes, spinal cord injury, pelvic fracture, chronic renal disease, ethanolism, multiple sclerosis, or genital trauma. The implant can be bent down easily and worn in a normal position under your clothing. It is a safe and successful cure for organic impotence.

A penile implant can improve your sex life, but it will not necessarily make you fertile. If you want to father a child, you should request a complete fertility workup before getting the implant. You should know your odds before undergoing surgery.

Premature Ejaculation

If you cannot control your ejaculatory responses for at least thirty seconds after penetrating your wife's vagina, you may suffer from premature ejaculation. Some prefer to broaden this clinical definition: if you cannot control your ejaculatory responses for a sufficient length of time to satisfy your partner at least half of the time, you have premature ejaculation.

Premature ejaculation becomes a fertility problem when you ejaculate prior to inserting your penis fully into your wife's vagina. Of course you can always consider artificial insemination with your sperm. However, given a choice, most couples prefer using "natural" techniques. You can often control this condition by changing coital position and by using a behavior modification procedure called the "squeeze technique."

The *squeeze technique* helps desensitize your penis so you can participate in sex without experiencing premature ejaculation. When using this procedure, your wife places her thumb on the frenulum on the underside of your penis. (See figure 8-2.) She places her first and second fingers on either side of the coronal ridge on the top of your penis. Squeezing her fingers together for three to four seconds in this manner will make you lose your urge to ejaculate. You may also lose some of your erection. After fifteen to thirty seconds your wife can stimulate your penis again and just before you ejaculate repeat the squeeze technique. If your wife is concerned about how much pressure to use, you can place your fingers over hers and press with her.

This demonstration of ejaculatory control improves your self-confidence and will be a major step toward reestablishing communication and improving your marital relations. Once you've practiced this technique, you can try it with her in the female-superior coital position (wife on top). After using the squeeze technique several times, she can insert your penis into her vagina *without* thrusting her pelvis to stimulate you. With counseling many couples are able to establish "normal" coital patterns and pregnancy.

Ejaculatory Incompetence

Men with this disorder rarely have difficulty achieving or maintaining an erection; however, they cannot ejaculate during sex. Often the wife is unaware of her husband's condition because he simulates orgasm. I can detect this problem by comparing the semen analysis with the postcoital test. If your semen test is normal but there are no sperm in the cervical mucus after sex, ejaculation did not occur. This rare psychological condition sometimes responds well to behavior therapy. Ejaculation may be stimulated by combining masturbation and manual stimulation with eventual insertion into the wife's vagina. If the condition persists, you can overcome the fertility problem by using AIH with a masturbated ejaculate.

Retrograde Ejaculation

Retrograde ejaculation is a condition in which semen is ejaculated into the bladder rather than out through the urethra, because the bladder sphincter does not close at the moment of ejaculation. It is found in 1.5 percent of infertile men and is the most common cause of absent ejaculate. If you have this disorder, you may notice that your ejaculate volume is small (below one milliliter) and that sometimes after intercourse your urine looks turbid or cloudy. The diagnosis can be confirmed by examining a urine specimen taken soon after intercourse. If large quantities of sperm are found in your urine, retrograde ejaculation is the fertility problem.

Retrograde ejaculation often occurs in diabetics, paraplegics, and men taking blood pressure medication (antihypertensives). The disorder may also occur in men with urethral stricture or men who have undergone surgical repair of their bladder, prostate, or other abdominal structures.

Many times medications such as decongestants, which contract the bladder sphincter, will control retrograde ejaculation. In certain circumstances, surgical reconstruction of the bladder neck can restore normal ejaculation. Consult with your doctor to see if you are a candidate for surgical intervention.

The most common fertility treatment method involves retrieving the sperm from the man's bladder and artificially inseminating his wife. This is the technique I tried with Michael and Shelley T. Since sperm cannot survive in an acid urine, I asked Michael to take one teaspoon of bicarbonate of soda in a glass of water four times a day for two days prior to Shelley's most fertile time of the month. About twenty minutes prior to collecting his semen, I asked Michael to empty his bladder. After he ejaculated into a jar, I catheterized Michael to collect his semen together with a small amount of urine. I then washed the sperm and using a syringe placed the sperm into Shelley's cervix.

The success rates are quite good, provided the couple can stick to the regimen. I told this couple that we'd need to repeat the procedure twice monthly until Shelley got pregnant. However, since Michael's religious beliefs made him reluctant to masturbate, they did not want to continue this procedure. So I recommended a less invasive sperm collection method.

I suggested they have sex when Michael had a full bladder. It seems that the weight of the urine on the bladder neck and/or increased sphincter squeezing may direct the semen into the penis instead of the bladder. I also told them to try to have sex with Michael standing upright. Michael and Shelley found this method much more to their liking. However, Shelley still did not conceive. We had some more work to do with Shelley's endometriosis. I'll discuss the procedures I used in a later chapter.

To avoid catheterization, I can also use the full bladder technique to collect a semen sample for AIH. If the man ejaculates very little semen, he collects the first five milliliters of his urine for washing and insemination. This technique will result in a 50 percent pregnancy rate.

Obtaining Semen Artificially

"Normal" ejaculation may not be possible for many men who are physically impaired; for example, if they are quadriplegic. However, semen can often be obtained by artificially stimulating the man to ejaculate. Using a vibrator to stimulate his penis is a simple and often effective technique. (Some of you may not even consider this to be "artificial.") When this fails, electrical stimulation will make half of these men ejaculate, and an additional 15 percent will have retrograde ejaculation. Thirty-five to 40 percent will not ejaculate because of the pain experienced from the procedure. It's possible, however, that many of these men could ejaculate under general anesthesia. Decisions about using these options should involve the couple and their physician.

Because male fertility has been shrouded in mystery, I've covered male fertility problems in much greater detail than most fertility books do. I hope that with the understanding you've gained in these chapters, you will be able to ensure that your physician is giving you the best opportunity to reach your fertility potential. When you and your wife *both* maximize your fertility, you have the best chance for getting your miracle baby.

III. Female Fertility

9. Female Fertility Problems: Clues from Your Past

"Doctor, I can't get pregnant!" Kathy's voice belied her controlled exterior. "We want a baby so badly. You're our last hope."

"Kathy," I said, glancing at her history form, "tell me when your periods stopped."

She sat straight and squared her shoulders. "Two years ago."

I scanned the page. "You're a runner. Do you enter the Tulsa Run?"

Her face brightened. "I wouldn't miss it. Last year I came in twelfth."

"That's very good. How long have you been running?"

"I really started training two years ago. Up to then I wasn't so serious about competing."

Two years ago, I thought. And two years ago her periods stopped. Now I had the first important clue to Kathy's fertility problem.

I knew she wouldn't like what I was about to suggest. "Kathy, we know that women athletes often complain that their periods stop. Of course, I need to know a lot more about *you,* but I wouldn't be surprised if your training regimen is contributing to your fertility problem."

Her smile faded. "You mean I'll have to stop running?"

"Not at all," I assured her. "Many women athletes keep in shape even while they are pregnant. But first, let's figure out how to *get* you pregnant."

She smiled. "Sounds good to me."

Physical exertion is only one of many factors that may affect your fertility. Critical points about your development, medical history, and life-style all give me vital clues to solving your fertility problem. In this chapter you'll learn what your doctor's investigations into your past can reveal, and gain insight into what may be causing your fertility problem.

Analyzing Your Life-style

Excessive or Rigorous Exercise

This cause of infertility may be grounded in our ancestral heritage. If food supplies were low, we followed herds of migrating animals or ranged far and wide to gather fruits and grain. A pregnancy would impair the woman's ability to keep up with the group. To improve her odds for survival during famine, nature decreased her fertility so that she stopped ovulating and her periods ceased (amenorrhea). This is probably the same protective mechanism that caused Kathy S.'s problem.

Fortunately, resolving Kathy's hormonal imbalance was easy once I identified the cause. I'll tell you how we treat amenorrhea in a later chapter.

Emotional Stress

Most women with fertility problems appear to be under a great deal of stress. But we don't know for any one person whether the stress contributed to the fertility problem, or whether the fertility problem brought on the stress. Many women in high stress situations become pregnant, so we can't say conclusively that stress will disrupt your hormonal balance.

We do know, however, that stress can affect your hypothalamus, the part of your brain that controls sex hormones. And we know that some women who have no apparent reason for being infertile except stress will often respond to a medication that improves hypothalamic function.

I'm not saying that the old wives' tale "Just relax and you'll get pregnant" will work. However, there's a great deal about the link between fertility and stress that we don't understand.

Dieting and Nutrition

Low calorie diets, special athletic diets, eating disorders, and other restrictive eating practices may impair your fertility. A number of factors may cause this problem: (1) losing the weight itself, (2) reaching a low percentage of body fat, (3) reaching an absolute minimum weight, (4) stressing the body, and/or (5) suffering from a nutritional imbalance. The mechanism for reducing your fertility isn't clear and it may vary from one individual to another. Like Kathy S., however, the most common complaint is amenorrhea, lack of menstrual periods. (I frequently find that teenagers who have been on crash diets stop having periods.)

Fortunately this is one of the easiest fertility problems to correct. When you change your diet and gain weight, you start ovulating and menstruation resumes.

Strangely enough, I've also seen ovulation stop in women who follow *strict vegetarian diets*. I remember one woman who ate so many carrots that her genitals turned bright orange. The stress of her diet and high blood levels of carotene (from eating carrots) may have caused her anovulation. Rather than taking medication to induce ovulation, she chose to cut down on her vegetables and add fish and eggs (protein) to her diet. Having thus increased her caloric and protein intake, she began ovulating and soon became pregnant.

Women weighing two hundred pounds or more may also have fertility problems. This may also be one of nature's protective mechanisms, since *obesity* does not provide the best environment for fetal development and birth. In fact, before the age of modern medicine, many obese women and their babies died in childbirth. Nature apparently prefers to reduce your fertility and wait for you to lose weight.

I remember one woman who, at five foot four and 188 pounds, complained of irregular periods with heavy flow. The reasons for her fertility problem are interesting. It seems that fat cells themselves can convert androgens (hormones produced by the adrenal gland) into estrogen (female hormone). Assessing all her symptoms, I suspected that her fat cells were producing enough estrogen to confuse her brain. Her brain, thinking that the *ovaries* were producing the estrogen, lowered her pituitary gland hormone production, which in turn led to anovulation. (You'll learn more about how these complex hormonal systems control your monthly cycles and fertility in the next chapter.)

Once I explained how this woman's obesity affected her fertility and general health, she was more than willing to start a diet. A well-planned weight-reduction diet and exercise program eventually restored her fertility. And since her "reduced" fat cells no longer produced excess estrogen, she got a bonus: her risk of developing endometrial cancer diminished, too.

Gathering Medical Clues

Pelvic and Reproductive Tract Surgery

Adhesions (scar tissue) inside the abdominal cavity caused by pelvic infections or abdominal surgery can impair fertility. I commonly find scar tissue in women who have had surgery for ruptured appendix, bowel repair, cesarean section, ectopic pregnancy, or the removal of an ovarian cyst. Twisting around the ovaries, fallopian tubes, and even the uterus, these inflexible webs of scar tissue restrict the natural mobility of these delicate organs.

Margaret B., for example, had a ruptured appendix when she was twenty-three. When I looked at her reproductive organs through the laparoscope (telescope), I found that her pelvic adhesions were so extensive they prevented her eggs from entering her fallopian tubes. I clipped and removed the tissue from around the organs so that Margaret's tubes could once again gently flex and coax the ova down the narrow passage toward the waiting sperm.

Scarring may also occur inside the uterus. Debbie W., for example, came to me about a year after having a D & C, saying, "Ever since my gynecologist scraped out my uterus, instead of having a period I just spot each month." When I looked into her uterus with a hysteroscope (small telescope), I found her uterine walls stuck to one another. I used a rather simple yet effective procedure to separate her uterine walls so they could heal and begin functioning normally. I'll discuss more about this procedure in a later chapter.

Frequent Vaginitis

If you suffer from frequent yeast or trichomonias infections, you may also have chlamydia, which can cause tubal damage. Because of increased exposure, women with a number of different sexual partners have a much greater chance of contracting these infections. A history of frequent vaginitis will alert me to the possibility that you have pelvic adhesions and tubal blockage. Once diagnosed, these abnormalities may respond to corrective surgery.

Illnesses May Impair Fertility

A number of illnesses can lead to impaired fertility. The most obvious ones are the venereal or *sexually transmitted diseases* such as gonorrhea, chlamydia, ureaplasma infection, and pelvic inflammatory disease (PID). These diseases can scar your uterus, block your tubes, and cause the formation of pelvic adhesions.

I remember one woman who said that four years ago her doctor thought she had a gallbladder problem. "I had a pain right here," she said, holding her hand over the lower right half of her rib cage. "I guess it just went away, because I haven't had any more trouble."

After asking her several questions about her symptoms I suspected that instead of having a gallbladder problem, she had probably contracted PID. After further tests, I discovered that PID had caused her liver to adhere to the inside of her abdominal wall, a condition called *Fitzhugh-Curtis syndrome.* Once I surgically removed the adhesions and repaired her scarred fallopian tubes, she soon became pregnant.

Other diseases such as *hepatitis (liver disease)* and *kidney disease* can cause fertility problems. Both your liver and kidneys filter and remove waste products, toxic substances, and impurities from your blood. A buildup of wastes and unmetabolized (not chemically broken down) hormones may interfere with your menstrual cycle. When these diseases are brought under control, fertility usually returns.

Thyroid gland disorders may also interfere with fertility. Increased metabolism from an overproduction of thyroid hormone (hyperthyroidism) will burn up your estrogen supply faster than your body can make it. Without estrogen you cannot ovulate. In contrast, if your thyroid gland produces insufficient thyroid hormone (hypothyroidism), you will stockpile too much estrogen and you may have an elevated prolactin level. If you have an excess of these two hormones, your ovaries cannot function normally. Regulating your thyroid production through surgery or thyroid supplements usually restores fertility.

Hypertension (high blood pressure) may be associated with an adrenal gland disorder that causes excessive production of male hormones (androgens). *Increased androgens* can disrupt normal ovarian function as well as disturb your female secondary sex characteristics.

I remember one woman referred to me for a fertility workup said, "Doctor, I'm growing a mustache!" The hair growth on her upper lip (a condition called hirsutism), very oily skin, and acne told me she was probably producing excessive androgens. As I expected, her blood tests revealed that she had an overactive adrenal gland. When she received medication to slow her androgen production down, her periods resumed, and much to her relief her mustache stopped growing.

Treatment for Abnormal Pap Smears

Cone biopsy, laser surgery, or cryosurgery may be used to treat a condition detected by an abnormal Pap smear. Any of these procedures can degrade the quality of your cervical mucus to the point that sperm cannot travel into your uterus. I performed a cone biopsy on a twenty-seven-year-old patient of mine who had a precancerous Pap smear result. I hoped I could halt the growth of abnormal tissues and prevent Nancy V. from developing cervical cancer. A year later she married and wanted to have a baby. When I performed a postcoital test, I found that her mucus was too scant and thick for the sperm to pass. So I recommended we wash her husband's sperm and inject them directly into her uterus (intrauterine artificial insemination homologous). After three tries Nancy became pregnant.

A cone biopsy can also weaken the cervix and allow premature pregnancy loss. So during Nancy V.'s pregnancy I watched her cervix to make sure that it stayed shut until delivery. Fortunately all went well and she delivered an eight-pound fourteen-ounce baby boy. I'll discuss more about the procedures I used with Nancy in chapter 19.

Anticancer Agents and Radiation

Anticancer agents such as methotrexate or radiation treatment may also compromise your fertility. Radiation can cause not only pelvic adhesions but also chromosomal damage to your eggs. If you're concerned about the effects of these treatments, talk with your doctor.

Endometriosis

Endometriosis may scar your fallopian tubes, interfere with your ability to ovulate, and prevent embryo implantation. Endometriosis is the presence of endometrial tissue outside the womb. Unfortunately we do not know the exact mechanism by which endometriosis forms. Being sensitive to monthly hormonal changes, this tissue grows and then, as does the endometrium in the uterus, sheds during menstruation. This "bleeding" inside the abdominal cavity is very painful, as Shelley T. testified: "When my period starts, my cramps get so bad I have to go to bed."

When I looked inside Shelley T.'s abdomen with a laparoscope, I found extensive pelvic inflammation and scarring. Since endometriosis can also cause tubal blockage, I injected dye into her uterus and tubes to see if they were open. I was really relieved to see the blue inklike fluid seeping out each fimbria (the opening of the fallopian tube near the ovary).

Fortunately endometriosis frequently responds to hormone therapy and, when necessary, to surgery. In Shelley's case I decided to use the laparoscope and a small instrument passed through a second small incision to cut her adhesions. Then I used a laser to selectively cauterize the endometrial implants. A later chapter will explain more about these procedures.

German Measles (Rubella)

German measles (rubella) does not impair fertility. However, if you contract rubella during the first half of your pregnancy, your baby will likely suffer from severe defects, including deafness and mental retardation. It would be tragic to undergo extensive fertility treatment only to achieve a pregnancy blighted by German measles. Therefore, I always do a blood test to determine if my fertility patient is immune to German measles. If the test is negative, I give her a rubella vaccine. I then recommend that the couple use barrier contraception, such as condoms, for three months to avoid the remote possibility that the live virus vaccine could affect their baby.

Tender Breasts and Milky Discharge

If your breasts are tender or if you have a milky discharge, you may have breast tumors. If I cannot detect any abnormal growths, I look for other factors that can cause a hormone imbalance—for example, an excess production of prolactin.

Prolactin, one of the primary hormones responsible for milk production (lactation), suppresses ovulation. I remember one patient who came to me because she hadn't responded to the drugs her doctor prescribed to induce her to ovulate. Heather P. complained of milk leaking from her breasts, so I suspected that her pituitary gland was producing excessive amounts of prolactin. When this was confirmed by a blood test, I prescribed Parlodel (bromocriptine), an oral medication. That did the trick and she got pregnant in her very next cycle. I'll discuss this treatment more in chapter 12.

Neurological Disorders

Any disturbance in your central nervous system may interrupt the delicate hormonal coordination between your hypothalamus, pituitary gland, and ovaries. If you suffer from seizures, epilepsy, visual disturbances, poor sense of smell, dizziness, loss of balance, or chronic headaches, you may have a neurological disorder. If you take medication to control epilepsy, nervous tension, depression, and so forth, the drugs themselves may interfere with your fertility. I remember one RESOLVE member who reported that when her doctor changed her antidepressant to a different prescription she began ovulating three months later. I may consult with a neurologist if I feel the disorder requires further diagnosis and treatment. Once we correct the neurological abnormality, fertility may return naturally.

Medications That Compromise Fertility

A number of medications may compromise your fertility. If you take hormones, antibiotics, or antihypertensives, they can prevent an embryo from implanting in your uterus. If taken in the middle of your menstrual cycle, Motrin, Anaprox, Indocin, or aspirin—usually taken to ease menstrual cramps—may prevent your ovary from releasing a ripened egg. Antidepressants, hallucinogens, painkillers, and alcohol may increase your prolactin levels and cause ovulation failure. When you stop these medications (and *don't* stop taking any medications without consulting your doctor first), fertility usually resumes.

Be sure to tell your doctor about every prescription or over-the-counter drug you take. These drugs may not only play a part in your fertility problem but, should you become pregnant, they may also jeopardize the development of your infant. My general rule of thumb is "When in doubt, do not take it." We honestly do not know the effects of all drugs on a pregnancy, particularly when taken in combination with other medications.

Illicit Drugs

Central nervous system depressants such as heroin or large, frequent doses of marijuana can interfere with your sex drive and with the hormonal balance necessary for ovulation and menstruation. Don't bother to pay for expensive fertility treatment if you plan to continue taking these drugs. Besides, during your pregnancy, a number of these drugs may also threaten your unborn child. Both marijuana and tobacco cigarettes increase the carbon monoxide level in your blood and impair your unborn baby's oxygen supply. Without adequate oxygen, tissues and vital organs may be damaged or killed. Taking hard drugs like cocaine will also reduce the life-sustaining blood supply to your unborn baby. When you stop using these toxic chemicals, your fertility usually returns.

Massive Hemorrhage During Childbirth

At a RESOLVE meeting I met a woman who had nearly died with the birth of her first child. During her delivery she had suffered a massive hemorrhage. "They gave me twelve blood transfusions," she reported. "My baby and I just barely survived." She picked up her infant and held her close. "I tried to nurse Rachael, but she was starving, so I gave it up. After a few weeks it was all I could do to get out of bed, feed her, and change her diapers."

Her husband interrupted. "I knew something had to be wrong, so I put Sarah and Rachael in the car and drove them to the doctor."

"The doctor told us that massive bleeding associated with pregnancy sometimes shocks the pituitary gland to the point that it dies," Sarah said. "He called it *Sheehan's syndrome*. He didn't know exactly why this happened to me, but my pituitary may have suffered a temporary loss of its blood supply."

Since Sarah's damaged pituitary gland no longer controlled her thyroid hormone production, adrenal hormone production, and blood sugar levels, she experienced a wide range of symptoms including extreme fatigue. In addition, she could not ovulate, she could not have a period, and she could not have another baby. When her doctor put Sarah on pituitary hormone replacement therapy, she eventually regained her fertility and gave birth to a second child.

Assessing Your Gynecological History

When Are You Most Fertile?

Day 1 of your menstrual period is *the day your period begins*. This seems relatively simple, but you wouldn't believe how many people fail to get pregnant because they count the days from the wrong starting point. (Just recently I spoke to a couple who counted from the day her period *stopped*. They knew she was most fertile around the middle of her cycle, or approximately days 14 to 16, so they timed intercourse two weeks after her period stopped. However, since her period stopped on what they should have counted as day 6, they were having sex a week too late—on days 20 to 22.)

Because on the average a woman's cycle varies in length from twenty-six to thirty-five days, you cannot count forward from day 1 to find your most fertile days. Since you ovulate approximately fourteen days *before* your next period begins, you count backward fourteen days from the date you expect your next period will start. That means the woman with a thirty-five-day cycle would ovulate on day 20 or 21 and the woman with a twenty-six-day cycle on day 11 or 12. Since you're fertile for only twenty-four hours each month, these calculations become quite critical.

I use a number of methods to determine the time of peak fertility, but many women, however, can do so by increasing their awareness about their bodies. Around the time of ovulation many women sense a discomfort on one side of their lower abdomen. The feeling associated with ovulation, called *mittle-schmerz,* does not occur in women who do not ovulate—for example, in women taking birth control pills. Also at the fertile time of the month women often notice a *clear stringy mucus discharge* from their vagina. When your mucus thins out, it allows sperm to swim through the cervical canal. This definitely signals the *right* time to have sex. I'll discuss other methods you can use to pinpoint your peak fertility in a later chapter.

Cramps and Pelvic Heaviness

If you have *cramps* or take medication for cramps, your doctor needs to know how severe they are. Severe pain at the onset of your period may indicate the presence of endometriosis. If you do not become bloated, do not cramp, and develop only a scanty flow, you may not be ovulating. That's why women who take birth control pills often have less discomfort during their periods. Fortunately ovulation induction treatment is successful for most women.

If you experience *pelvic heaviness,* you may have large fibroids (noncancerous growths) in your pelvis. Fibroids may also interfere with your ability to conceive and with the ability of your uterus to support an early pregnancy. When necessary, the offending fibroids can be surgically removed and fertility restored.

Menstrual Flow

A *heavy monthly flow* may indicate that too-persistent estrogen production is overstimulating the growth of your uterine lining. A *scanty flow* may indicate that your body produces too little estrogen to prepare the uterine lining for implantation, or that you have intrauterine adhesions. When estrogen levels are controlled, normal menstrual flow resumes and the quality of the uterine lining improves. When indicated, intrauterine adhesions can be surgically removed.

Spotting during the middle of your cycle may indicate a hormonal imbalance or abnormalities inside your uterus—for example, the presence of scar tissue or an IUD you forgot about. Don't laugh. I once removed an IUD from a patient who had tried to get pregnant for two years. When I extracted the coil she'd received some four years earlier, she was shocked, saying, "But my doctor said I'd passed it!" When the string disappeared, her doctor assumed her uterus had expelled the IUD. In fact, her uterus had "swal-lowed" the string and concealed its presence for two years. Never assume.

Amenorrhea

"Doctor, I'm not having monthly periods. My husband and I want a baby. What should I do?"

When I hear this complaint, I first establish whether the woman has *ever* had a period. If she has, then her reproductive tract is patent (intact and open to the outside). If she has never menstruated (primary amenorrhea), I examine her to determine if she has a uterus, if her uterus opens into a vagina, and if the vagina opens to the outside. If the vaginal tract is closed, I can open it surgically and restore fertility. However, if her reproductive organs are missing or severely deformed, not much can be done to correct the abnormal-ities. If her ovaries are intact, new technologies provide hope that her eggs can be fertilized and nurtured in another woman's uterus. (See "Hysterec-tomy" below.) If I've established that she is not pregnant and has no physical abnormalities, I begin to look for signs of hormonal deficiencies.

Secondary amenorrhea, or the cessation of periods after they've been initiated, is a much more common finding. Secondary amenorrhea may be caused by pregnancy, damaged uterine lining, ovulatory failure, ovarian failure, hypothalamic failure, or pituitary failure. First I determine if your hormonal systems are functioning properly. For example, if your breasts are underdeveloped, if your pubic hair is absent or scanty, or if you have signs of virilization such as a mustache (hirsutism) or masculinized genitalia, I'll suspect a hormone imbalance. If I find elevated FSH (pituitary hormone) levels, I'll suspect ovarian failure. (Remember, this is also the sign for testicular failure in men.) Only by performing a complete fertility workup can I identify the reason for your failure to menstruate. Hormone stimulation and replacement therapies are successful in most of these cases.

Because amenorrhea is the most common complaint of women with fertil-ity problems, I've devoted chapters 12, 13, and 14 to discussing ovulatory failure and treatment.

D&C

If you've had a D&C (dilation and curettage) to scrape out the contents of your uterus, the doctor treating your fertility problem needs to know why. Sometimes a doctor performs a D&C to remove unwanted scar tissue or the remains of an incomplete abortion. Instead of the D&C improving the uterine environment as expected, however, sometimes the procedure will cause the inflamed uterine walls to stick (adhere) together. People with *Asherman's syndrome,* as this condition is known, usually have *regularly occurring, scanty periods.* I can correct this condition with a rather simple procedure described in chapter 19.

Traumatic Abortion

If a trained physician using sterile procedures performs your abortion, you do not need to worry about compromising your fertility. Illegal, back-alley, and self-induced abortions may lead to life-threatening infection and tubal blockage. Damage to your cervix from a traumatic abortion may also increase your risk for early pregnancy loss. Fortunately these complications occur must less frequently since the Supreme Court legalized abortion.

Spontaneous Abortion and Miscarriage

I need to know if you've ever been pregnant, if you've had an elective abortion, or if you've carried a baby to term. A previous pregnancy demonstrates to me that at some point in your life you were fertile. If your present husband fathered a child with you, I know even more—that *together* you were fertile. That's a very important piece of information, since there is clear evidence that *your fertility potential depends on a unique compatibility between you and your partner.*

I also need to know if you lost a baby early in a pregnancy. The positive side of a spontaneous abortion or an ectopic pregnancy is that you *can* get pregnant. The reactions to early pregnancy loss, however, are anything but positive. The couple suffers shock, disbelief, anger, sadness, and grief.

Many women may discard a developing embryo within the first month or so of pregnancy without realizing it. Researchers therefore believe that the spontaneous-abortion rate may be as high as 25 percent. However, if a woman reports *repeated abortions,* I will want to assess if her uterine lining can support a pregnancy and if her cervix will remain closed throughout the pregnancy. I'll discuss more about correcting these problems in chapter 19.

Ectopic Pregnancy

If scar tissue blocks the pencil-lead-sized fallopian tube passage (lumen), the tiny sperm may be able to get through but the larger, dividing fertilized egg may get stuck. Entrapped by adhesions, the embryo implants in the tube and continues to grow.

Damage to the inside surface of the tube may also interrupt the fertilized egg's journey to your uterus. Waving like blowing grass, the tiny hairlike cells (cilia) lining the inside of a normal fallopian tube stroke the fertilized egg toward your uterus. When infection or surgery strips the cilia from the walls of your tube, the immobilized embryo may attach itself to the smooth tubal wall.

Unfortunately the condition that damaged one of your tubes very likely damaged your other tube. For this reason, if you have one ectopic pregnancy, you have an increased chance for another one on the opposite side. Years ago women suffering from an ectopic pregnancy often lost the affected fallopian tube. The job of creating another pregnancy fell almost exclusively to the remaining ovary and tube. Now, however, with early pregnancy detection and microsurgery, we can often save the affected tube and restore it to a functional state.

In the next few chapters I will reveal many more of nature's fascinating secrets and tell you how you can overcome and cope with pregnancy losses.

Did Your Mother Have a Fertility Problem?

Quite frequently fertility problems run in families. Therefore, clues from your mother's past may help me unravel a complex mystery. I remember a thirty-year-old woman who came to me after she'd had two miscarriages. She told me her mother had also miscarried twice before giving birth to her. I asked my patient to find out if, in order to avoid another miscarriage, her mother had taken a drug called DES when my patient was in utero. We were both greatly relieved to find out that her mother had not taken this insidious drug. Had she been exposed to DES, my patient could have suffered from unexplained infertility and repeated unexplained pregnancy losses, as well as have a deformed cervix and womb.

Congenital Uterine Abnormalities

Congenital abnormalities of the female genital tract range from a simple septum dividing the uterus in half to a complete duplication of all structures— uterus, cervix, vagina, and external genitalia. Some of these abnormalities may interfere with implantation of the embryo or lead to early pregnancy loss. Surgical correction often improves the chances for maintaining a pregnancy to term. Sometimes endometriosis can cause a tipped uterus. The tipped uterus, however, is not causing the fertility problem; the endometriosis is.

Hysterectomy

Today women who had previously given up hope of pregnancy because of a hysterectomy may be able to have their own babies. Using in vitro fertilization techniques, we can surgically retrieve her eggs and fertilize them with her husband's sperm. Since she cannot carry the pregnancy, we deposit the fertilized embryo into a surrogate (substitute) mother's womb. Though born to another woman, the baby will carry its true parents' genes. These exciting prospects are medically possible, and the legal system is grappling with the issues they raise. I'll tell you more about these techniques in chapter 21.

Contraceptives and Infertility

Sexual Freedom

Modern contraception, usually regarded as a great success story, may actually be responsible for dramatically increasing fertility problems. The upside of contraception is that women can enjoy sex and still avoid unwanted pregnancies. With the ability to control their fertility and plan their lives, women are making remarkable progress in the educational, artistic, and business worlds. And with the fear of unwanted pregnancy removed, many women enjoy sex with different men. They're glad to see the demise of the double standard.

The unfortunate downside to freely available contraception is that liberated sex has given rise to a rampant increase in sexually transmitted diseases. Every year over 250,000 college-aged women become infertile from chlamydial infection alone. And many of them won't know it until some years later. Whereas women in the past feared unwanted pregnancy, they should now fear pelvic inflammatory disease. I offer no easy answers for the man or woman who wants a free sex life. We do know that barrier contraceptives such as condoms and diaphragms lower your risk of contracting sexually transmitted infections. My hope is that medical breakthroughs will provide a vaccine or some other means for curbing this epidemic.

The IUD

The IUD, or intrauterine device, particularly exposes the woman to an increased risk of pelvic inflammatory disease and tubal damage. Although the exact mechanism of contraception is not well understood, the IUD apparently creates a low level inflammation which prevents the embryo from implanting in the uterus. Acting like a wick, the IUD string may allow bacteria from your vagina to enter your womb, where they can flourish and invade your delicate reproductive structures. There's some evidence, though, that copper IUDs may offer some protection against infection.

Since the risk of contracting a sexually transmitted disease and impairing fertility increases with exposure to different partners, the IUD has been removed from the American market. I have asked all my patients who use IUDs to have them removed if they plan to have children.

The Pill

Using the Pill won't impair your fertility; however, its use may disguise an underlying fertility problem. I remember when Shelley T. approached me in a panic:

"God's punishing me! I know it!"

"Birth control pills did not *cause* your fertility problem, Shelley." Once she calmed down a bit I asked, "What were your periods like before you took the Pill?"

"I had terrible cramps," she told me. "But the Pill changed that."

"The Pill may have reduced your cramping, but it did not cure your endometriosis. It's been with you all along," I told her.

The Pill may also artificially regulate women who normally have irregular periods. When their irregular cycle returns after they go off the Pill, these women are often surprised. All the time they took the Pill, they falsely assumed that it had cured their underlying hormone imbalance. It is true that up to 3 percent of women using the Pill will develop menstrual irregularities as a direct result. However, they usually respond very well to ovulation induction therapy. I'll discuss more about the Pill in chapter 12.

Lost Years Lower Your Odds

Couples who use any contraceptive method over a prolonged period of time have only a few remaining fertile years in which to resolve their fertility problem. To compound the difficulty, their fertility naturally declines as they grow older. However, since women can manage a healthy pregnancy through their late thirties, these couples succeed quite frequently. They just need to pursue their fertility treatment more aggressively.

Sexual Practices

Lubricants and Contraceptive Creams

A lubricant used during sex may contain spermicidal chemicals that attack and kill millions of sperm before they have a chance to enter the protective cervical mucus. Even petroleum jelly may interfere with sperm activity. The easiest and cheapest lubricant is your own saliva, although bacteria in your mouth may degrade the semen. I suggest that if necessary my patients use a water-based lubricant such as K-Y Jelly or Lubrifax. If you're in doubt about what product to use, ask your doctor.

Douches

If you douche before having sex, you may alter the environment in your vagina and deteriorate the quality of your mucus. Later, when the sperm arrive, your vaginal passage may be hostile and your cervix blocked by mucus that sperm cannot penetrate. If you want to make a baby, I do not recommend douching before sex.

Even though most sperm penetrate your mucus within a couple of minutes of ejaculation, I recommend waiting at least thirty minutes after sex before douching. Actually, unless you have some personal preference for douching, you *never* need to douche regularly. I'm amazed by the ability of commercial advertisers to make money from our fears about smelling bad or being dirty.

Timing

If you don't have sex, you can't get pregnant. You can quote me on that. You'd be surprised at the number of people who do not have sex the national average of two and one-half times a week. You are fertile for about twenty-four hours each menstrual cycle and sperm can survive in your reproductive tract for twenty-four to forty-eight hours. So you can see that if you do not have sex every forty-eight hours around the middle of your cycle (during your fertile days), you probably will not get pregnant.

Many factors can interfere with sex—the couple may be too busy, the husband and wife may travel, they may be under too much stress. During fertility treatment you may need to reduce your activities, alter your business schedules, and even cancel vacations. It doesn't make much sense to spend $300 to $500 in a month to become fertile and then blow your chances because of a trip.

Too Much Sex

You know what they say about too much of a good thing. . . . Seriously, though, extremely frequent sex reduces the amount of sperm available for each ejaculate. We know that it takes about forty-eight hours after sex for a man to build up an adequate supply of sperm. So having sex more frequently than that reduces the man's sperm count so much that pregnancy becomes even less likely. So you'll just have to control yourself—at least until you get pregnant.

Uncomfortable or Painful Sex

Uncomfortable or painful sex may indicate infection or other abnormalities. Sometimes, however, discomfort may only be due to insufficient lubrication. If your vagina is consistently dry during sex, perhaps you and your husband should engage in foreplay longer. Stimulating your nipples, clitoris, and other erogenous areas will make your glands secrete natural juices. If your vagina remains dry after sexual arousal, your lubricant-supplying glands may be infected or your hormones may be deficient. You may require low-dose estrogens to improve your vaginal secretions or you may choose to use a water-soluble lubricant. You need to discuss this problem with your doctor.

Aversion to Sex

Sometimes sex turns a person off. One particularly sad case comes to mind where, as a child, my patient had been sexually abused by her uncle. To Donna N. sex was shameful and to be avoided as much as possible, even though she loved her husband.

After she told me about her uncle and her abortion at age thirteen, I referred her for counseling. Although it took some time, her relationship improved to the point where she looked forward to pursuing fertility treatment. If sex turns you off, seek professional advice.

Your Fertility Treatment History

Many couples who come to me already have completed all or part of a fertility workup. They may have been referred to me by their doctor or perhaps they became discouraged and wanted a second opinion. Often they are surprised when I tell them I may need to repeat many of their tests. However, there are a number of factors I must consider:

Often the reports I receive for previous tests do not contain all the information I need for proper interpretation. For example, only when I know both the test date and the ovulation date can I evaluate your postcoital test and biopsy results.

I know and trust my assistants, technicians, and the outside laboratories I use. Due to the lack of standard methodology, many medical laboratories do not check for ureaplasma infection or do not do a good job of reporting sperm morphology on a semen analysis. I remember one instance where a couple came to me after the wife had undergone fertility treatment for over a year. When I repeated the husband's semen analysis, I found ureaplasma. Four months after I treated them with antibiotics, she became pregnant. Since I'm responsible for my patient's care, I want the best information I know how to get.

While conducting a pelvic exam, I make many observations that may not be noted on your previous physician's report. I notice, for example, how easily I can manipulate your pelvic organs. If they are stiff and rigid, I may suspect adhesions. Subtle clues like flinching when I touch your ovary or kicking when I do your rectal exam help me solve the mystery. I'll also find out if your condition has improved or grown worse since your previous doctor examined you.

I need to perform X rays and/or laparoscopies so I myself can view the dye moving through your tubes. The written results of a previous laparoscopy do not tell the whole story. Watching the flow and the response of your reproductive organs to manipulation tells me much more, for example, than knowing that you have a tubal blockage. If necessary, I can even lay out a specific plan for performing corrective surgery. I'll discuss the use of diagnostic laparoscopies and X rays in much more detail in later chapters.

People change with time—for better and for worse. Your fertility potential one year ago is history. I must assess your *current* condition before I can design a customized treatment plan.

When you change doctors, bring your old records on your first visit and, if possible, also bring your hospital records and X rays. By providing these records, you may not totally avoid the need for duplicating tests, but you'll minimize your expense and you'll give your doctor an edge on solving your fertility problem.

Your doctor should use every available clue from your past because considering every factor will give you the best chance for having your miracle baby.

10. Unraveling Your Fertility Mystery

When an Agatha Christie mystery begins to unfold, at first the investigator suspects every character of having committed the crime. As the plot unwinds, however, our hero gradually pieces together one shred of evidence after another, until, in the final climactic scene, the master investigator pinpoints the culprit.

There's little difference between conducting this kind of investigation and doing a fertility evaluation. When a woman first comes to my office, I suspect a broad range of causes: tubal blockage, endometriosis, pelvic adhesions, uterine abnormalities, anovulation, and so forth. As I review her history, I search for clues that will help me narrow my list of suspects. Repeated pelvic infections, for example, lead me to suspect tubal blockage or pelvic adhesions. If she tells me she's not menstruating, I'll focus my investigation on hormonal problems or uterine abnormalities. If she complains of extreme discomfort when her period starts, endometriosis will be uppermost in my thoughts.

Just as the master detective can be thrown off by misleading evidence, I must also be cautious not to jump to conclusions. It's all too easy to say, "Pain at menstrual onset? You have endometriosis." Although this may be correct, endometriosis may not be the only offender. Intrauterine adhesions or hormonal imbalances may also play a part.

The challenge presented by contradictory clues can seem overwhelming. Just as I think I'm about to close in on one suspect, I uncover evidence that doesn't seem to fit the pattern. With my theory blown out of the water, I must formulate a new strategy for tracking down the culprit. By analyzing the clues and continually searching for additional ones, I draw closer and closer to the solution until I reach the climactic day when I tell you that you are pregnant.

Lucy H., for example, had infrequent periods and pain with intercourse. Ovulation induction therapy had regulated her periods but she'd failed to get pregnant. When her doctor referred her to me, I performed a laparoscopy (telescopic examination of the inside of her pelvis) and discovered that she had endometriosis and that adhesions (scar tissue) encased her ovaries. Even if she had ovulated, her eggs could not have reached her fallopian tubes.

The Six Female Fertility Factors

The six key elements of female fertility are:

1. Ovulation
2. Sperm-mucus interaction
3. Fertilization
4. Tubal transport
5. Embryo implantation
6. Miscarriage

During the physical examination and fertility workup, I attempt to confirm or eliminate each of these candidates as hinderances to your fertility. Your history may point strongly to some of them. The clues I gather during the physical examination will offer additional evidence. Once I've pinpointed the areas of greatest concern, I can recommend specific tests and procedures to confirm my diagnosis. For now, though, I'd like to discuss what clues I can gather from the physical examination. Please refer to figure 10-1 as I discuss this subject.

The Physical Examination

During the physical examination I look for evidence that you are ovulating, that your mucus allows sperm to reach the egg in good shape, and that the fertilized egg can successfully implant and grow in your uterus. A number of things may go wrong during this process. The sperm may not be able to journey through inhospitable cervical mucus or, having reached the egg, they may be unable to penetrate its surface. The egg may get lost in the body cavity and never find its way into the fallopian tube. Fallopian tubes, damaged by infection or trapped in adhesions, may not be capable of moving the egg toward the uterus. The growing, fertilized egg may become entangled in webs of intratubal adhesions caused by infection and develop into an ectopic pregnancy. Or the uterine lining may fail to nourish the early embryo. Once I determine where these processes are breaking down, I have a good chance of restoring your fertility.

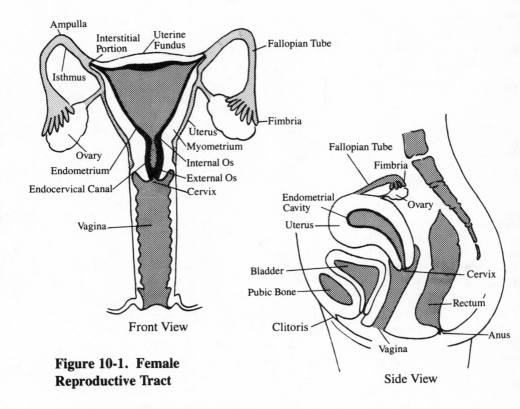

**Figure 10-1. Female
Reproductive Tract**

Fertility Factor #1: Ovulation

Any woman who comes to me complaining of very heavy menstrual flow, very light menstrual flow, no menstrual flow, irregular cycles, breast discharge, or scanty or overabundant body hair growth is telling me that she may not be ovulating. This may be due to an intrinsic malfunction of her reproductive organs or hormones, or to a systemic disease causing other body chemistry problems.

During the physical examination I look for evidence of systemic disease: jaundiced (yellow) skin and eyes are indicative of liver disease; tenderness in the middle of the back and water retention (edema) may indicate kidney malfunction.

Nancy F., for example, had been trying to get pregnant for six months. When I examined her, I found that her ankles and fingers were swollen. Further tests indicated that her kidneys were not functioning well. I referred her to a kidney specialist, since once her kidney function improved, her periods would probably return to normal.

Since your liver and kidneys filter impurities from your blood (including "old" hormones), their function is vital for maintaining hormonal balance. If

I find high blood pressure together with excessive body hair, I may suspect adrenal gland abnormalities, which can affect ovarian function. (I discuss more about how we diagnose and correct these problems in the chapters on ovulation.)

I also look for other clues pointing to ovulation problems. For example, if you weigh over two hundred pounds, if you're severely underweight, or if you have a highly developed athletic build, I may suspect a hormonal imbalance. Kathy S., who ran fifteen to twenty miles a week, had leg muscles a man would be proud of. It didn't take much imagination to know that she was exercising to the point that she would cause ovulatory failure. (Chapter 9 explains the mechanisms for these disorders.)

When I examined Dorothy L., I found that her thyroid gland was swollen, and she appeared lethargic. Suspecting a thyroid deficiency, I ordered a thyroid hormone blood test. After she began taking a thyroid supplement, she became more energetic, had much more interest in having sex with her husband, and her periods returned to normal. Five months later she called to tell me she was pregnant.

Both hyperthyroidism (overproduction of thyroid hormone) and hypothyroidism (underproduction) may interfere with your menstrual cycle by disturbing estrogen supplies. I'll discuss more about how your hormonal system works in chapters 11, 12, and 13.

When I examined Gale P., I found that she had a translucent, white discharge from her breasts. She said that she'd had a milky discharge ever since she'd stopped nursing her toddler. I suspected she was producing excess prolactin, a hormone usually associated with nursing mothers. This hormone prevents ovulation and pregnancy so that you can give your baby the best nutrition possible. When you're trying to get pregnant, however, you don't need prolactin's birth control protection. With treatment, Gale's fertility quickly returned.

Your body build and secondary sex characteristics may provide additional clues to hormonal imbalance. Undersized breasts, scanty pubic hair, and underdeveloped hips all suggest a female hormone deficiency. An enlarged clitoris and abnormal hair growth such as a mustache may suggest excess male hormones. Rarer conditions such as ambiguous genitalia (not clearly male or female) and duplicate reproductive organs may point to genetic or enzyme defects that can interfere with ovulation. Although breast size, body conformation, and hair distribution are not conclusive evidence, they may corroborate suspicions created by other clues.

If your menstrual history and evidence from your physical examination point to ovulatory problems, I will recommend a number of tests to confirm this diagnosis. Like the detective, I need corroborative evidence to prove my case. Chapters 11 through 14 describe in detail what can cause ovulatory problems and how, with treatment, most women with ovulatory disorders can get their miracle babies.

Fertility Factor #2: Sperm-Mucus Interaction

Normally your cervical mucus forms an impervious plug that keeps foreign materials, including sperm, from entering the uterus. Once each month, responding to estrogen, the cervical mucus becomes clear, thin, and stringy so sperm can swim through the cervix into the uterus.

I'll examine your cervix to make sure that the mucus has not been degraded by infection, by a cone biopsy to remove abnormal precancerous tissue, by cryosurgery, or by cervical deformities from congenital defects or DES exposure (as in Debbie W.'s cervix). In part IV, "When Sperm Meets Egg," I'll explain how I diagnose and treat sperm-mucus problems.

Since bacteria, viruses, white blood cells, and antibodies may attack and impair the sperm, a number of different vaginal and cervical infections can cause fertility problems. Some wave red flags in the form of pus (purulent discharge), inflammation, itching, burning, and foul odors, but many of the more insidious varieties can be detected only by special laboratory tests.

Minor infections include candidiasis or yeast, which may be uncomfortable and itchy; trichomoniasis, which may produce a bad-smelling greenish discharge; gardnerella infection, which causes a burning sensation and a gray, pasty discharge; and ureaplasma infection, which is symptomless. A microscopic examination of the discharge will disclose the identity of the invading organism. Once antibiotics eradicate these infections, fertility may improve.

Infections such as chlamydia, ureaplasma, and gonorrhea occasionally cause severe illness leading to tubal blockage and the formation of adhesions, often without the victim knowing it. Diagnosis is difficult, since the only evidence may be a reddened vagina or a burning sensation and urgency to urinate. In the presence of an abnormal cervical discharge, I will test for all of these organisms.

Janice D.'s laparoscopy, for example, revealed that she had extensive pelvic adhesions. When I questioned her, the only incident she could recall was a flulike illness she'd had during her junior year at college. She and her physician had never realized she was suffering from a chlamydia infection. It was six years later, when she couldn't get pregnant, that she received the diagnosis.

By causing an inflammation of the uterine lining, ureaplasma (often called mycoplasma) may lead to early miscarriage. When this sexually transmitted infection is found in the woman, it will probably be in her partner, too. When ureaplasma occurs in the man, he may form antibodies which attack his own sperm. Since the symptoms for this disease are as elusive as those for chlamydia, only a culture can help me diagnose it.

Gonorrhea is usually symptomless in the woman, although in some cases it causes a bad-smelling yellowish discharge and red and swollen vaginal walls, and if it invades your tubes, you'll suffer severe pain and develop a high fever. In the presence of infertility I always culture for this organism because, once detected, I can often restore fertility with the antiobiotic doxycycline.

During the vaginal examination I will also note if you appear to be having an abnormally high level of discomfort. This sometimes indicates psychological problems which could interfere with having intercourse. Since you are fertile for only forty-eight hours each month and sperm survive for only forty-eight hours in your reproductive tract, infrequent intercourse may play a role in your fertility problem.

Fertility Factor #3: Fertilization

Fertilization depends on the sperm's ability to penetrate the outer layers of the egg and transfer its genetic information. Since I cannot determine if fertilization is working properly from the physical examination, I must use the sperm penetration assay or the acrosin test, which are explained in chapter 18.

Fertility Factor #4: Tubal Transport

Other clues uncovered during the physical examination may point to transport problems. Abdominal scars, for example, could indicate that surgery might have caused adhesions to form. Margaret B. had an appendectomy scar from a ruptured appendix. Since the massive infection and surgery could have caused tubal blockage, I did a tubal X ray right away.

Abdominal adhesions can prevent the egg from entering the fallopian tube as well as impede its passage through the tube. I have seen many women whose tubes were frozen in place by this nonstretchable tissue preventing the tubal movement necessary to coax the egg toward the uterus. During the pelvic examination I manipulate your reproductive organs to detect if they move freely or if they feel like rigid, plaster models. I can often restore fertility to women with adhesions by surgically removing this scar tissue. I'll discuss these procedures in chapters 16 and 17.

Wincing, tenderness, and pain during the pelvic examination may indicate an active infection, endometriosis, ovarian cysts, tumors, adhesions, fibroids (leiomyomata), or bladder infection. If your ovaries are enlarged or tender, I'll suspect an infection or that you're ovulating irregularly.

Endometriosis can cause adhesions and impair ovulation. Sometimes I can detect endometriosis during the vaginal and rectal examination; however, just as Sherlock Holmes pulled out his magnifying glass to get a closer view of the evidence, I often must confirm the diagnosis with a laparoscopy. When I examined Shelley T., I could feel the tell-tale beading or bumps on the surface of her reproductive organs and supporting uterine ligaments, but I followed up with a laparoscopy to confirm my diagnosis. Endometriosis may respond to medication or, failing that, surgery. I'll discuss more about endometriosis in chapter 17.

Depending on their size and location, fibroids and ovarian cysts can also interfere with egg transport. These conditions will usually respond to surgery.

Remember that having open tubes isn't the whole answer. If infection has stripped the hairlike cilia from the tubal lining, the egg may not be able to complete its journey toward the uterus. Detecting tubal problems during the physical examination is very unlikely; only an X ray can confirm that diagnosis. By combining the clues from your history and from the physical examination, I can decide if sperm/egg transportation might be contributing to your problem. A complete discussion of testing and procedures for tubal transport problems appears in chapters 16 and 17.

Fertility Factors #5 and #6: Embryo Implantation and Miscarriage

Sometimes during the physical examination I detect obvious causes for miscarriage such as congenitally malformed reproductive organs, an abnormally shaped cervix evident of DES exposure, or a cervix distorted by previous surgical procedures. Most of the time, however, the physical examination will not reveal the exact causes for recurrent miscarriage. The tests specific to this and other disorders causing pregnancy loss are covered in complete detail in chapters 18 and 19.

Standard Laboratory Tests

As part of the physical examination, I order a number of laboratory tests. Table 10-1 profiles the ones I use and what they tell me.

The Postevaluation Conference

The postevaluation conference I have with my patients reminds me of the meeting between the chief of detectives and his team to plan the final strategy for solving the mystery. Step by step the chief outlines the plan, so each person knows exactly how to play out his or her role. He also outlines contingency plans to deal with obstacles and unexpected events. And even with all this forethought and effort, sometimes the suspect isn't where they expect him to be; sometimes the suspect escapes; and sometimes the suspect turns out to be innocent.

As "chief of detectives," once I have collected all the clues from my investigation—your history, your physical examination, and your laboratory tests—I begin to outline a strategy for treating your fertility problem. I may not know the exact cause of your infertility, but I can customize the investigation to uncover the most likely problem. If I suspect ovulatory

Table 10-1
Laboratory Tests I Often Perform
During the Initial Workup

Cultures: Cultures for sexually transmitted infections reveal the presence of active infections which must be treated prior to initiating other fertility treatment. It's mandatory that the woman's partner be treated for the same infection, since bacteria are easily passed back and forth between sexual partners.

VDRL: This test rules out the presence of syphilis, which may affect the fetus as well as pose a serious health hazard to you.

Pap Smear: Although not specific to fertility problems, a Pap smear should be performed during every workup to eliminate the possibility that you have or may soon develop cancer of the reproductive organs.

CBC: A complete blood count will give a reading on your general health. It will also indicate if you have an infection, systemic disease, or iron deficiency.

Urinalysis: This test will help rule out renal disease or genitourinary tract infections as potential fertility problems.

Prolactin: This test should be done if you have a clear or milky breast discharge.

Thyroid Hormone: I run this test if the physical exam suggests hyper- or hypothyroidism.

Sed Rate: The sedimentation rate in your blood will often reveal an infection when cultures show up negative.

Rubella Titre: I always test for immunity to German measles, since contracting this disease during a pregnancy often leads to severe deformities in the fetus.

Semen Analysis: Your workup is not complete until your husband's semen has been evaluated. Performing extensive testing and treatment on you will be to no avail if he is not contributing adequate sperm.

---

problems, as I did with Kathy S., I will want to evaluate the menstrual cycle. If I suspect tubal blockage, as I did with Margaret B., I will order an X ray. If I suspect an infection, I'll recommend antibiotic therapy. Or if I find poor semen quality, I'll want to evaluate your husband more thoroughly. As I get closer and closer to the answer, I begin to put together my strategy for eliminating your fertility problem.

You as a couple are part of my assault team. Without your input, understanding, and participation, my efforts will fail. You will decide how much of your resources you are willing or able to spend, and how long you want to pursue your goal. Together we'll decide how aggressively to attack the problem. Margaret and Richard B. knew that due to Margaret's age they had only a few fertile years left. They had good insurance coverage, so they wanted to check everything out as soon as possible, with money as no object. Shelley and Michael T., in contrast, had already been through a year or more of tests, had many bills to pay, and Michael was feeling so pressured that he was ready to quit entirely. They chose to proceed more slowly—one step at a time. The fertility treatment plan we worked out for these two couples differed considerably.

To help you understand the types of decisions you may be facing, the next chapters will cover specific tests and treatments for the six main suspects in female infertility.

11. Are You Ovulating?
Clues from
Your Menstrual History

The complexities of regulating ovulation remind me of the difficulty a musical conductor faces when combining a hundred individual performances into a symphony. Although each individual plays an important part in the production, the overall performance ultimately depends on the precise *coordination* of all the players. If even one instrument is unsynchronized or off-key, the delicately balanced harmony can turn into disorganized noise.

In the "ovulation symphony" harmony can be disrupted by disturbances in the menstrual cycle. Instead of an unwavering pattern repeated from month to month, infertile women frequently complain that their periods are irregular or have stopped altogether, and some women have never experienced menstrual flow.

So, like the semen analysis, your menstrual history serves as a simple screening test to guide my investigations. It won't tell me precisely what the fertility problem is, but it will tell me where to look for further clues.

The Three Types of Menstrual Patterns

The Regular Menstrual Period

The critical point about this category is that your period is *regular* from month to month, beginning like clockwork every twenty-five days or every thirty-five days, for example. If your periods are regular, you are probably ovulating. The *consistently irregular* menstrual cycle, however, where one month you begin menstruating after twenty-five days, the next month after thirty-four, and the next in thirty, may indicate that you have a fertility problem. If a woman reports a regular menstrual history, I'll usually look at other areas of the reproductive system for a breakdown in the fertility formula.

Irregular Menstrual Periods or Amenorrhea for Six or More Months

This is the most common complaint found with fertility problems. The woman's menstrual periods occur infrequently and at unpredictable intervals. Some women, like Kathy S., even report that at some point their periods stopped altogether. Because these women are capable of menstruating (as demonstrated by their history), there is a good chance that with the proper treatment ovulation and a regular menstrual cycle will resume.

Nonexistence of the Menstrual Period

Women who have never menstruated may have genetic abnormalities, congenitally deformed reproductive organs, delayed puberty, or a pituitary malfunction. If by the age of sixteen a woman has not started menstruating, she should be concerned. It is important to diagnose the problem early and to determine if such women will respond to hormonal therapy or surgical correction. The emerging new technologies offer the most promise to these people. More about that in chapter 21.

What Is Ovulation?

Ovulation is a fascinating harmony performed by several different "players"—your hypothalamus, your pituitary gland, and your ovary. Your hypothalamus maintains the hormonal "tempo" by regularly pulsing GnRH (gonadotropic-releasing hormone). These pulses stimulate your pituitary gland to produce LH (luteinizing hormone) and FSH (follicle-stimulating hormone). (See figure 11-1.)

Your pituitary gland plays the chorus—a pattern repeated from month to month in a beautifully precise rhythm. Each month the pituitary secretes FSH to stimulate the development and growth of over one thousand eggs. This phase in the ovulation cycle is known as the follicular phase. At puberty a woman has about half a million primitive germ cells. Only four or five hundred, however, will ever reach maturity. Due to some mysterious mechanism which we don't yet understand, usually each month only one of the thousand developing eggs becomes dominant and grows to maturity. This egg, or ovum, is cradled within the ovary in a tiny, fluid-filled capsule called the *follicle*.

During the follicular phase of your cycle, LH acts on the ovary's theca cells to initiate estrogen production by the granulosa cells. (See figure 11-1.) The estrogen makes the follicle even more responsive to FSH, which further stimulates follicular growth and development of the egg. As the follicle expands toward the surface of the ovary, the egg increases in size nearly forty times. The ovary tells the pituitary when it needs more or less FSH to finish

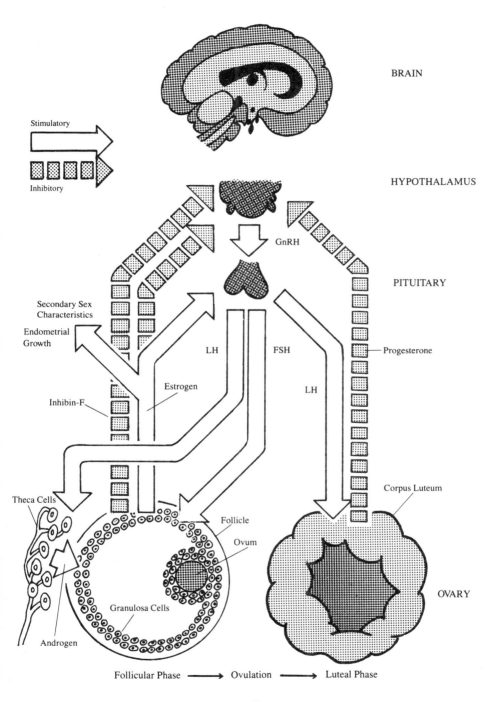

Figure 11-1. The Female Hormone System

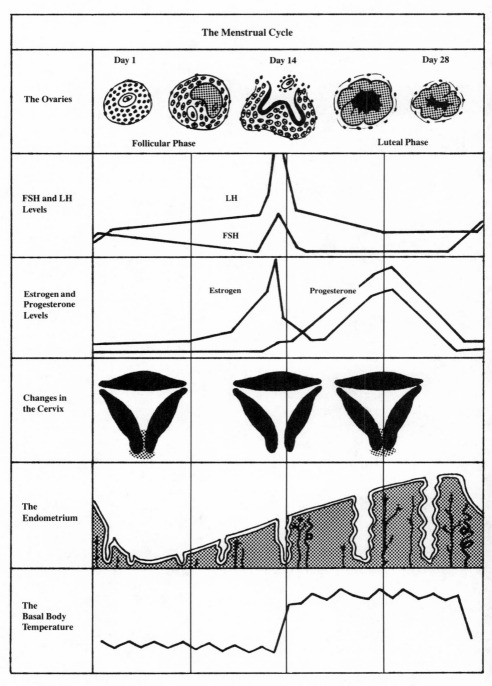

Figure 11-2. Cyclical Changes in the Menstrual Cycle

the job of egg maturation by making a feedback hormone called inhibin-F (folliculostatin).

Shortly before ovulation, the genetic material (nucleus) in the egg divides (meiosis) to half the number of chromosomes in the cell. If the egg is fertilized, a second meiotic division leaves the ovum with twenty-three chromosomes—a perfect complement to the sperm's twenty-three. To form an egg, the female germinal cell divides twice, as does the male germinal cell. During female germ cell divisions, however, the "surviving" ovum jealously hoards the bulk of cellular material (nutrients) and casts off the excess genetic material (polar bodies). The egg or (if the egg is fertilized) the embryo survives on these nutrients until the embryo successfully implants in the woman's uterus.

Estrogen also stimulates the uterine lining (endometrium) to become thick, lush, and filled with nutrients for the embryo. The cervical mucus responds to elevated estrogen by becoming clear, watery, and stringy. Normally impervious to sperm, at midcycle the mucus welcomes the sperm and promises easy passage toward the egg. When dried on a slide, the "friendly" mucus shows a characteristic ferning pattern. (See figure 15-2 on page 160.)

When your estrogen level peaks at midcycle, the pituitary "knows" that the egg is ready to embark on its journey. The pituitary responds to the estrogen peak by producing a surge of LH, which releases the egg within eighteen to thirty-six hours. The outer wall of the ovary dissolves away from the bulging follicle, and within two to three minutes the ovum escapes into the woman's abdominal cavity. Surrounded by a sticky protective layer of cells (cumulus oophorus), the egg gently floats toward the fallopian tube. The expelled follicular fluid stimulates the fimbriated end of the fallopian tube to reach toward the ovum, grasp the ovary, and vacuum up the egg. The muscles and tiny hairs (cilia) lining the fallopian tube gently coax the egg on its three-to-four-day journey through the narrow passage. For conception to occur during this cycle, the sperm must fertilize the egg in the fallopian tube within twelve hours of ovulation. (See figures 10-1 and 15-1.)

During the egg's journey, the ruptured follicle begins an amazing transformation into the corpus luteum. Stimulated by LH from the pituitary gland, this yellow-pigmented, glandular, ovarian structure enlarges to make up nearly a third of the ovary. During the *luteal phase* (latter half of the cycle), the corpus luteum produces progesterone, a hormone that prepares the uterine lining for implantation of the embryo. Progesterone also acts on your body's temperature-regulating mechanism by raising basal body temperature (BBT) approximately one-half degree. Thus shortly after ovulation, you will see a rise on your BBT chart.

If fertilization does not take place, the corpus luteum deteriorates. Estrogen and progesterone levels decline rapidly in the week or so prior to menstruation. Deprived of these hormones, the endometrium atrophies and menstrual flow begins. At the site of the original follicle the corpus luteum degenerates and leaves a minute piece of scar tissue as a reminder of its brief existence.

If fertilization takes place, a *corpus luteum of pregnancy* forms to maintain the uterine lining (endometrial bed) and support the implanted fertilized ovum (conceptus). I'll discuss more about fertilization and implantation in chapter 19.

The hypothalamus, pituitary, and ovary must all work in perfect harmony. When they do not, the most obvious symptom is abnormal menses. And the nature of the abnormality clues me into the source of the problem. Table 12-5, "Conditions That Can Interfere with Ovulation and Menstruation," gives an overview of which fertility problems are caused by malfunctions of the hypothalamus, pituitary, ovary, pituitary feedback system, and other related systems. The diagnosis and treatment for these disorders are discussed in the remainder of this chapter and in chapters 12 and 13.

In the remainder of this chapter I will explain how I approach evaluating ovulation in the woman with a regular cycle. The next two chapters will explain how I approach evaluating women who have never had a period and women who have irregular periods or periods that have stopped.

Evaluating the Woman with Normal Menstrual Periods

"My period is so regular," Margaret B. explained, "that whether or not I've started, on the thirtieth day I insert a tampon before I go to work. By noon I'm always glad I did, because otherwise I would have had an accident."

When I hear this type of menstrual history, I'm almost certain that the woman is ovulating each month. My attention turns immediately to diagnosing other fertility problems. However, on the outside chance that nature is tricking us into complacency, I ask the woman to keep a basal body temperature (BBT) chart for a couple of months. When accurately kept, the BBT will confirm the timing of ovulation and will help me properly schedule other tests.

Interpreting the Basal Body Temperature Chart

The normal ovulatory pattern: Measure your basal (resting) body temperature first thing in the morning—even before getting out of bed. During the follicular phase (the first half of your cycle) the "normal" BBT pattern should show only slight variations in your temperature (under 98 degrees). In response to progesterone produced at midcycle by the corpus luteum, your BBT will rise about a half degree (to about 98.4) and should remain elevated until your next period begins. The two or three days *preceding* the temperature elevation are your most fertile. After your temperature rises, the odds of initiating a pregnancy become minimal. By reviewing this data over two to three months, you can usually predict your most fertile days.

Failure to ovulate: If your temperature remains relatively constant throughout your cycle, you did not ovulate.

Short luteal phase: If you are undergoing ovulation induction treatment, you will want to pay particular attention to the fourteen days following ovulation. Should your period start within ten days of the temperature rise, you may have a progesterone deficiency (luteal phase defect). Without an adequate progesterone supply the uterine lining will not develop properly and the embryo will fail to thrive.

Sustained temperature rise: A sustained rise in your temperature—beyond the date for your next period—should make you jump for joy because you are probably pregnant!

Additional data: Variations in temperature levels aren't the only data recorded on BBT charts. You can also indicate the days you menstruate (with an X), the days you have sex, the day you feel mittleschmerz (the twinge of pain associated with ovulation), and days when you are ill or out of sorts. Figure 11-3 shows a sample BBT chart. When kept with care, this record can provide valuable information for planning your fertility treatment. Table 11-1 explains how to keep your chart.

Don't get too uptight about keeping the BBT chart. If doing so causes you problems, discuss it with your doctor. Although the BBT can provide important supportive data, it isn't absolutely necessary. Your peace of mind is far more important than creating a graphic history of your sex and reproductive life. Although a serum progesterone test indicates whether you have ovulated, it does not help pinpoint the day of ovulation.

Taking an Endometrial Biopsy

By examining a tiny piece of uterine tissue, I can evaluate how well prepared your uterus is to accept an embryo. I use the BBT and your menstrual history to time the biopsy one to three days before your next period begins.

With one rare exception (where the egg remains trapped in the follicle, a condition called luteinized unruptured follicle), a normal endometrial biopsy confirms that you are ovulating, that you have an adequate luteal phase, and that your uterine environment will support an embryo. I'll discuss more about the endometrial biopsy in chapter 19.

If a woman's menstrual cycle appears normal, I proceed down different diagnostic paths. However, if any of these test results look suspicious, I treat her as I would a woman with abnormal menstrual periods. Read on to learn how I diagnose menstrual abnormalities.

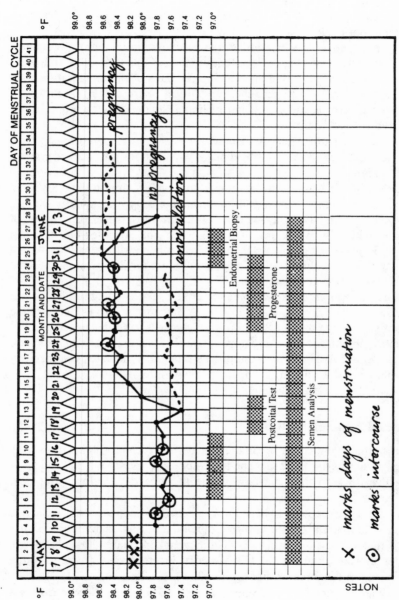

Figure 11-3. Basal Body Temperatures and Timing for Tests

Table 11-1
How to Keep
Your Basal Body Temperature Chart

1. Begin taking your temperature on the morning your menstrual period ends.

2. Shake down the thermometer the night before and place it on a bedside table.

3. At your first waking moment take your temperature by inserting the thermometer in your mouth, vagina, or rectum for five minutes. Do not vary your procedure from day to day or month to month. Use a clock to time yourself. DO NOT smoke a cigarette, eat or drink, or get up to go to the bathroom or to go find your thermometer before taking your temperature.

4. Record the *thermometer reading* on your chart under the correct day of your cycle (day 1 is the first day of your period). Record the *days you have sex* by placing an arrow at the bottom of the column. Record the *days of your menstrual flow* with an X. Record *mittleschmerz* if you feel it. *Note any exceptions* on your chart—for example, if you are ill, did not get a good night's sleep, or are running a fever. Also mark when your doctor performs any tests and what they are.

5. Wash the thermometer with cool soapy water, rinse it, shake it down, and place it in its protective case beside your bed. Some people prefer to use alcohol or disposable plastic thermometer protectors.

6. Repeat this procedure every day until your next period begins. Each month start taking your temperature on the morning your menstrual period ends.

7. Take your charts to every doctor's appointment.

Living with BBT

Keeping the BBT chart is an inexpensive method for observing your menstrual cycle and hormonal system at work and an indirect method for pinpointing ovulation. BBT charts will help indicate your most fertile days, so you can plan sex at the "right" time of the month.

I've had some women tell me in total frustration that they're ready to flush their thermometer down the toilet. "If I have to plot another flat line, I think I'll scream. Every morning the mercury reminds me that I'm a failure."

I have a few suggestions that may help you put BBT charting into proper perspective:

1. Think of taking your temperature like brushing your teeth: you do it without even thinking. The BBT is more convenient because you don't even have to get out of bed to do it.

2. Make BBT charting into a game. See which one of you can guess the day that your temperature will rise. The one who wins gets taken out to eat (at the other's expense, of course!).

3. If you are the analytical type, use your calculator or personal computer to calculate median temperature during the follicular phase, percent difference to the luteal phase, and standard deviations. Where else could you find so much data to analyze?

4. Compare BBT charts at your fertility support group meetings. Award ribbons for those with the flattest line, for those with the highest midcycle temperature rise, and for those couples who had sex even during their infertile days.

Regular Menstrual Periods: Diagnostic Approaches Used to Determine If You Are Ovulating

Basal body temperature (BBT)
Serum progesterone
Endometrial biopsy

12. Finding Out Why Your Periods Are Abnormal

The two critical facts I need to know about a fertility patient who is having irregular or absent periods are (1) Can you menstruate? and (2) Can you ovulate?

Once I've answered these questions, I have a good idea of what's causing your fertility problem.

I'd like to share this information with you, as well as some of the questions and concerns my patients have brought up from time to time.

What Makes You Have a Period?

Normally each month estrogen and progesterone stimulate the growth of the uterine lining. When the progesterone-producing corpus luteum deteriorates toward the end of the cycle, "progesterone withdrawal bleeding" occurs: you have a period. Waves of vasoconstriction (blood vessel spasms) restrict the blood supply to the endometrium and thus provoke the onset of menses. At the conclusion of menses, clotting factors seal off exposed bleeding sites, and resumed estrogen production begins restoring the endometrium.

Initial Tests

Several basic tests will help determine why your periods are abnormal. Table 12-1, "Diagnostic Approaches for Irregular Menstrual Periods or Amenorrhea," which appears later in this chapter, will give you an overview of the diagnostic approaches used to determine if you are ovulating and the conditions that can interfere with ovulation and menses.

Pregnancy Test

This may seem surprising, but pregnancy is the single most common reason for women reporting to me that their periods have stopped. Before I initiate any type of fertility treatment, I conduct a pregnancy test to rule out the possibility of pregnancy.

Cervical Mucus Smear

Normally the cervical mucus is thick and relatively impervious to the outer environment. Throughout the first half of the cycle, increasing amounts of estrogen produced by the ovary cause the mucus to "fern." When placed on a slide and dried, the estrogen-primed mucus crystals form a beautiful fernlike pattern. Around the time of ovulation, high estrogen levels transform the mucus into a clear, watery, viscous fluid that sperm can easily transverse. After ovulation progesterone from the corpus luteum "opposes" the action of the estrogen, and the mucus once again thickens. I use this simple test to tell me if you've ovulated during this cycle. If you have not yet ovulated, I will observe the telltale ferning. I will then perform the progesterone withdrawal test to find out if you are capable of menstruating.

Progesterone Withdrawal Test

The progesterone withdrawal test will confirm if your uterus is capable of menstruating. If it is, then the cause of your menstrual irregularity lies with your hormonal systems. If your uterus cannot "bleed," then the problem lies with the uterus itself.

I can bring on your period either by giving you oral progesterone over a five- or ten-day period or by giving you a progesterone injection. After taking the progesterone, your period should begin within fourteen to twenty days. I prefer using the injection even though women often complain of a day of localized soreness. This cuts ten days of pill-taking off the waiting process.

Positive Response to Progesterone Withdrawal

If progesterone withdrawal causes your period to start up, as it did with Kathy S., I learn a number of things.

First, I know that your ovaries are producing enough estrogen to build up your uterine lining. I also know that your uterus is capable of responding to estrogen and progesterone stimulation. Since your uterus is functioning normally, your fertility problem lies somewhere in your hormonal system.

Second, you are failing to menstruate because you are failing to ovulate. For some reason your pituitary is not producing the LH spike necessary to release the ovum from your follicle.

Two conditions must exist before your pituitary will release an LH surge: The follicles growing in your ovaries must release enough estrogen to signal your pituitary that it's time to release the LH surge—in other words, that at least one egg has reached maturity. And your pituitary gland must be capable of generating the LH spike.

I may suspect that your hypothalamus just isn't prodding your pituitary well enough. If your follicles do not grow to maturity, you'll never produce enough estrogen to trigger the LH spike to release the egg and thus ovulate. A pituitary malfunction can cause the same problem; however, in Kathy's case, I suspected a hypothalamic insufficiency from excess running.

"How can you be sure?" Kathy asked.

"Well, that's exactly what my next series of tests will show. I want to make sure that other systems in your body are not adversely affecting your hormonal system."

Negative Response to Progesterone Withdrawal: Repeating the Progesterone Withdrawal After Estrogen Stimulation

Like Kathy, most women will "bleed" in response to progesterone withdrawal. However, if you don't, it's possible that your estrogen supply is not adequate to stimulate uterine lining growth. If your uterus is normal, taking estrogen to prime the growth of the uterine lining should guarantee that you'll have a period after progesterone withdrawal. So we'll try it again—this time giving you estrogen before the progesterone, just to be sure.

If the estrogen/progesterone-stimulated cycle fails to produce a "bleed," it means that your uterus cannot respond to estrogen and progesterone stimulation: we've pinpointed your uterus as the problem. My next step will be to examine the inside of your uterus. (I'll discuss uterine abnormalities, hysteroscopy, D&C, and uterine X-ray procedures in chapters 16 and 19.)

Positive Withdrawal to Estrogen/Progesterone Stimulation

When you have a period after taking estrogen and progesterone, I know that your uterus is capable of menstruating. The reason you have not been menstruating is that your ovaries are not producing adequate amounts of estrogen. At this stage in the diagnostic procedures we don't know for certain why your ovaries are not producing estrogen, but several possibilities exist: (1) your ovaries are not capable of producing estrogen, (2) your hypothalamus is not stimulating your pituitary to release FSH and LH, which control follicular development and estrogen production, (3) your pituitary is unable to produce adequate amounts of LH and FSH, (4) other hormonal imbalances are tricking your pituitary into "thinking" that it's doing a good job when, in fact, it is not.

Since estrogen stimulation is vital for the growth of the uterine lining, I will measure your estrogen hormone levels to confirm this diagnosis before venturing into new diagnostic territories. I'll also do a cytology smear to look at estrogen stimulation of your vaginal cells. In addition, I'll measure your FSH level to rule out ovarian failure. (A high FSH level indicates that the ovaries have been severely damaged or have run out of eggs.)

Detecting Ovarian Failure

Ovarian failure occurs when your ovaries are severely damaged or when they run out of eggs. When this happens, your pituitary gland tries to force your ovary to manufacture estrogen and to ovulate by working overtime to produce FSH. The pituitary gland's signals fall on deaf ears, though, because the damaged ovaries cannot respond to the extra FSH stimulation.

Ovarian failure may be caused by a number of conditions including infection, chemical toxins, medications, radiation exposure, tumor, and genetic abnormalities. Unfortunately ovarian failure is rarely reversible. However, ovarian failure due to infection or endometriosis will sometimes respond to treatment. Since a diagnosis of ovarian failure can be distressing, I always repeat the FSH test before recommending adoption or other alternatives.

Diagnosing Anovulation

Once we've ruled out uterine abnormalities and ovarian failure, we've confirmed that your periods are irregular because you are not ovulating (anovulation). For some reason your pituitary is not sending adequate amounts of LH and FSH to your ovaries. However, I have good news: the failure to ovulate, which affects 25 percent of infertile women, responds very well to treatment.

Symptoms of Anovulation

Although a few anovulatory women will have normal periods, most will have few or no periods at all (amenorrhea). Prolonged or heavy periods (menorrhagia), spotting during the middle of the cycle (metrorrhagia), and prolonged spotting may also occur. Women with anovulatory menstrual periods do not experience the typical menstrual discomforts often found in ovulatory women: breast soreness, mood changes, or cramping. The anovulatory woman's BBT chart will be flat (monophasic) and her cervical mucus will fern, indicating that progesterone (produced by the corpus luteum that forms after ovulation) never opposes the estrogen stimulation.

Tests Used to Determine the Cause of Anovulation

In the next phase of testing I try to determine why your pituitary gland is not stimulating your ovaries to ovulate. I need to answer a number of questions:

- Is your hypothalamus not "beating the drum" by producing regular pulses of GnRH?
- Is your pituitary gland damaged?
- Is your pituitary gland getting misleading feedback messages about ovarian function?

Several tests will give me the additional answers I need. Tables 12-1, "Diagnostic Approaches for Irregular Menstrual Periods
or Amenorrhea," and 12-2, "Hormonal Tests for Diagnosing the Cause of Anovulation," profile which tests I may order.

Table 12-1
Diagnostic Approaches for Irregular Menstrual Periods or Amenorrhea

Diagnostic Approaches Used to Determine If You Are Ovulating
Pregnancy test
Basal body temperature (BBT)
Cervical mucus smear
Progesterone withdrawal
    If progesterone withdrawal *does not* result in a period:
    Administer estrogen and repeat progesterone withdrawal
    If estrogen/progesterone withdrawal *does* result in a period:
    Cytology smear (to look at estrogen stimulation of vaginal cells)
    Estrogen blood test
    FSH test (if not elevated, may indicate pituitary or hypothalamic failure)
    If estrogen/progesterone withdrawal *does not* result in a period:
    Hysteroscopy (telescopic exam of uterine interior)
    Hysterosalpingogram (uterine X ray)
    FSH test (if elevated, may indicate ovarian failure due to genetic abnormality; may perform chromosome analysis)

Table 12-2
Hormonal Tests for Diagnosing the Cause of Anovulation

Prolactin Pituitary Hormone
Excessive prolactin can suppress pituitary output (LH and FSH) and can act directly on the ovary to suppress follicular growth.

Thyroid Hormone

Hyper- and hypothyroidism can interfere with hormonal metabolism (the rate at which hormones are used up by the body) and with the delicate hormonal balance between the pituitary and ovary. In addition, through an intriguing mechanism (explained later) hypothyroidism may contribute to excess prolactin production.

FSH and LH Pituitary Hormones

Elevated FSH almost always indicates ovarian failure. If FSH and LH are depressed, I suspect one of three things: that a faulty hormonal feedback mechanism is inappropriately telling the pituitary to cut back production; that the hypothalamus is not "beating the drum" to stimulate the pituitary to function; or that a pituitary inadequacy prevents the gland from functioning normally.

Adrenal Androgens (DHEAS and Testosterone)

In the presence of excessive hair (hirsutism) or male secondary sex characteristics (enlarged clitoris or ambiguous genitalia), elevated male hormone (testosterone), elevated DHEAS, or elevated adrenal androgens may indicate a congenital enzymatic defect, polycystic ovaries, or a tumor in the pituitary gland, adrenal gland, or ovary. Testosterone or adrenal androgens can suppress ovulation as well as cause a number of other problems discussed later.

Solving the Mystery of Anovulation

Twenty percent of ovulation failures result from stress, obesity, diet, excessive androgen production, thyroid gland dysfunction, or excess prolactin.

In the sections that follow, I will explain how these conditions can be identified and treated to resolve fertility problems. Chapter 14 describes ovulation induction treatment, which I may use if you have idiopathic anovulation (unknown cause) and which I may also use with some of the conditions discussed below.

Coming Off the Pill

Let me lay one fear to rest. It's very unlikely that oral contraceptives cause amenorrhea or anovulation. Oh, but you say, when you stopped the Pill, your periods never returned. Or perhaps they returned but were irregular and spotty.

To that I must ask, "What were your periods like before you took the Pill?" Usually the answer is "My periods were irregular. But I've had regular periods ever since I began taking the Pill."

So what's happening? Oral contraceptives do suppress ovulation; however, your uterine lining continues to cycle between development and shedding. Can you guess why you have a period? You may already know that the Pill contains estrogen and progesterone. When you stop taking the Pill for one week each month, you experience estrogen and progesterone withdrawal, and so you begin to menstruate. Something else happens that's also logical. You don't cramp, you don't bloat, and you don't become depressed—and that's because you don't ovulate. (Women who do cramp and bloat on the Pill may have other problems, which should be discussed with their physician.)

Each year thousands of women go off the Pill, and within two to four months they begin ovulating. If it is their goal, they soon become pregnant. However, a few women stop the Pill and resume an abnormal menstrual pattern, which may indicate that they are not ovulating.

For some it's possible that a fertility problem arose while they were taking the Pill. The cyclical action of the Pill may have masked the symptoms (menstrual irregularities) until they stopped taking it. This is why some doctors recommend that you stop taking the Pill for a few months every couple of years: to see if everything is still working normally. I do not recommend this practice, however, since one frequent side effect of this procedure is pregnancy. To me it does not make any more sense to go off the Pill every couple of years than to stop using condoms to see if you can still get pregnant.

The few women who do become anovulatory as a direct result of using the Pill usually respond very well to ovulation induction treatment with Serophene. (Chapter 14 describes how Serophene can be used to restore ovulation.)

Hypothalamic Malfunction

We suspect that a number of conditions may adversely affect hypothalamic performance: emotional stress, endorphins (nature's painkillers, which are synthesized by the brain in response to stress and pain), extreme exercise (amenorrhea athletica), dieting, poor nutrition, weight loss, low body fat, anorexia, and drugs, toxins, or medications. I discussed many of these conditions in chapter 9.

We cannot directly measure hypothalamic performance: we don't know for sure if the drum is beating. Sometimes, though, we can measure the *results* of insufficient hypothalamic stimulation. For example, we can test for low LH, FSH, and estrogen levels as described in table 12-2. However, often the changes are too subtle to detect.

Except for estrogen, the test results for Kathy S., for example, were all normal. When I discovered this finding, I had to assume that, as a result of her excessive running (stress), Kathy's hypothalamus was not pulsing GnRH in a manner sufficient to stimulate her pituitary. As a result, her pituitary was not properly stimulating follicular growth, her ovaries did not produce enough estrogen, and she did not ovulate. When I prescribed Serophene to enhance her hypothalamic activity, she began to ovulate. You'll learn more about Kathy's experience with ovulation induction in chapter 14.

Pituitary Gland Malfunction

Hormones from the pituitary gland control a number of "chemical factories" throughout your body: your adrenal gland, your thyroid gland, and your ovaries, to mention a few. When your putuitary malfunctions, many different systems can break down. The single most common end result, however, is an excess production of prolactin (hyperprolactinemia).

Hyperprolactinemia

Nearly 10 percent of women with irregular periods and 20 percent of women with no obvious cause for amenorrhea have elevated prolactin levels. One-third of these women may have a milky discharge from their breasts (galactorrhea) and one-third of them will have a pituitary tumor (adenoma). Almost always benign, these tumors respond well to drug therapy (bromocriptine) and to surgery. You may wish to refer to table 12-3, "Factors Causing Elevated Prolactin Levels," for an overview.

Excessive Exercise, Stress, or Suckling

Excessive stress and/or exercise may cause hyperprolactinemia. In addition, nursing a baby will release prolactin, nature's birth control hormone. When you stop nursing, relieve the source of your stress, or take Parlodel (bromocriptine), your prolactin levels will drop and ovulation will return.

Hypothyroidism

When your thyroid hormone production drops below normal, an intriguing chemical process leads to excess prolactin. Your hypothalamus also controls thyroid hormone levels by producing TRH (thyroid-releasing hormone), which tells your pituitary to make TSH (thyroid-stimulating hormone). When your thyroid gland cannot respond to these chemical signals, your hypothalamus senses that there isn't enough thyroid hormone around, so it produces more TRH, saying, "Get to work. We need more thyroid hormone."

Due to a unique chemical association, TRH also tells your pituitary to release more prolactin. The excess prolactin not only interferes with pituitary function but also exerts a direct inhibitory effect on the ovary itself. Taking a thyroid supplement to quiet your hypothalamus will usually correct this chemical imbalance and restore ovulation.

Elevated Adrenal Androgens (DHEAS)

We also find elevated adrenal androgens (male hormones) in one-third of women with excess prolactin. I'll discuss how these hormones can interfere with ovulation in the section on hormonal feedback below.

Severe Kidney Disease

Severe kidney disease, which impairs the body's ability to purify and filter the blood, may also result in the buildup of prolactin hormone. Dialysis, kidney transplants, or better management of the kidney disease may restore fertility to these women. The discussion on hepatorenal disease below will tell more about managing this disorder.

Medications

Certain medications may increase prolactin levels: phenothiazines and other tranquilizers; tricyclic antidepressants; methyldopa (Aldomet, an antihypertensive); Reserpine (antihypertensive); and narcotics. When these drugs are withdrawn, prolactin levels will return to normal. If you are concerned about a particular medication that you are taking, discuss it with your doctor.

Table 12-3
Factors Causing Elevated Prolactin Levels

Neurologic	Suckling
	Stress
	Hypothyroidism
Metabolic	Exercise
	Kidney failure
Medications	Phenothiazines and other tranquilizers
	Tricyclic antidepressants
	Methyldopa (Aldomet, antihypertensive)
	Reserpine (antihypertensive)
	Narcotics
Excess Androgens	Polycystic ovary
	Adrenal disease
	Congenital adrenal hyperplasia
Pituitary	Prolactin-secreting tumor
	Empty sella syndrome
	Growth hormone secreting tumor

Treatment for Hyperprolactinemia

The nature of your treatment depends on the cause of the elevated prolactin. Table 12-4, "Treatment for Hyperprolactinemia," explains a number of treatment options. Except for obvious systemic problems such as thyroid inadequacy and kidney failure, I usually prescribe Parlodel (bromocriptine) to lower prolactin levels. Parlodel will also reduce pituitary tumor size, should one be present. An oral medication taken with meals, Parlodel has few side effects, is relatively inexpensive, and—should you get pregnant—will not adversely affect your baby. Women with hyperprolactinemia respond well to this medication and their fertility usually returns quite quickly.

Table 12-4
Treatment for Hyperprolactinemia

Cause	Treatment
Pituitary tumor	Parlodel (bromocriptine) Surgery/X-ray therapy
Thyroid insufficiency	Thyroid hormone supplement
Adrenal androgen excess	Parlodel Cortisol Surgery/X-ray therapy
Kidney failure	Kidney transplant Dialysis
Empty sella syndrome	Parlodel
Medication	Terminate or change medication
Idiopathic (unknown)	Parlodel

Pituitary Gland Failure

Damaged Pituitary Gland

If your pituitary gland has been damaged by surgery, tumor, radiation therapy, and/or excessive bleeding during childbirth (Sheehan's syndrome), it may not be able to produce LH and FSH hormones in adequate amounts. To restore function to your ovaries, and your fertility, I must replace these hormones. Pergonal (LH and FSH) is the most common medication used for this purpose. (See chapter 14.)

Cushing's Disease

Though rare, Cushing's disease is characterized by elevated growth hormone (ACTH) secreted from a pituitary tumor. If you have this disease, you will have excess androgens (male hormones) and possibly excess prolactin (found in 20 percent of women with Cushing's disease). This condition can often be corrected by surgically removing the pituitary tumor.

Empty Sella Syndrome

Empty sella syndrome occurs when spinal fluid leaks into the bony chamber (fossa) housing your pituitary gland. Empty sella syndrome may happen because of a congenital weakness, surgery, trauma, or a pituitary tumor. When pressure from the spinal fluid compresses the pituitary gland against the bony walls of the fossa, you may lose LH- and FSH-producing cells, and you may lose your fertility. Lowering your prolactin levels with Parlodel (bromocriptine) and supplementing your LH and FSH levels with Pergonal (LH and FSH) should correct your fertility problem.

Hormonal Feedback Problems Affecting Your Pituitary Gland

Many systems in your body can trick your pituitary gland into producing fewer ovarian stimulants. Like production supervisors, your hypothalamus and pituitary gland monitor ovarian performance by sensing levels of estrogen and other chemicals circulating in your blood. In this way the pituitary knows when to speed up or slow down ovarian production. However, when other hormones get out of balance, the feedback messages from your ovaries become distorted and your hypothalamus and pituitary gland respond inappropriately. When this happens, your periods become irregular and you stop ovulating.

Hepatorenal Disease

Hepatorenal diseases affect your body's ability to filter impurities from your blood. Both your liver *(hepato-)* and your kidneys *(-renal)* remove toxins and "old" hormones from your system. If estrogen or adrenal androgens (see discussion of adrenal disease below) are allowed to build up in your blood, they tell the pituitary, "Stop stimulating the ovaries. Don't send out any more LH and FSH." The hypothalamus mistakenly thinks that your elevated estrogen supply is coming from ripening follicles. When the pituitary reponds to this message by slowing down FSH production, your immature follicles fail to develop and you stop ovulating.

If you have this problem, artificial blood filtration methods such as dialysis may not be adequate to restore your fertility. Pregnancy may not be advisable, however, since it may place an undue strain on your already compromised physical condition. Once your physician arrests the disease and the filtration systems work, your fertility will return.

Adrenal Disease (DHEAS)

Adrenal diseases usually cause two feedback problems: both excess adrenal androgens and, in 30 percent of these cases, excess prolactin (see above) will lower LH and FSH production and cause anovulation. Several different conditions may contribute to DHEAS elevation:

- Psychological or physical stress
- Pituitary, ovarian, or adrenal tumors
- Congenital adrenal hyperplasia (an inherited disorder)

Fortunately 30 to 40 percent of the women having mild DHEAS elevation will respond to ovulation induction therapy, without my having to treat the basic cause of the DHEAS elevation. If your prolactin hormone is also elevated, Parlodel will reduce both your prolactin and androgen levels.

Women with high androgen levels will show signs of virilization, such as growing a mustache (hirsutism). In these cases I must find out what's causing the elevated androgens and treat this condition. Elevated adrenal androgens are associated with Cushing's syndrome, congenital adrenal hyperplasia, or polycystic ovaries.

Cushing's Syndrome

Cushing's syndrome, another rare disorder, can be identified by the presence of "buffalo hump" (characteristic lump of excess fat located between the shoulder blades), water retention (edema), high blood pressure (hypertension), obesity, weakness, bruising, moon face, acne, hirsutism, and menstrual dysfunction. If you have these classic symptoms, I'll run a test to determine if you have an androgen-secreting tumor. If you do not have a tumor, low-dose cortisol medication will get your adrenal androgen production under control, and your fertility will return. If the test shows you do have a tumor, surgical removal of the tumor will restore your ability to ovulate.

Congenital Adrenal Hyperplasia

The classic symptoms of congenital adrenal hyperplasia include significant androgen excess, excessive hair growth, and an enlarged clitoris (clitoromegaly). If you have this inherited disorder, you may be shorter than your peers and you may have a family history of this disease.

Because of an enzyme deficiency, you cannot make cortisol. So the chemicals that your body normally uses to synthesize cortisol build up, and your body uses them to make androgens. The excess levels of androgens suppress ovulation. I can treat this disorder by supplementing your cortisol supply. When I replace your missing hormone, you will stop pumping out the chemicals to make cortisol and your androgen levels will return to normal. When this happens, you will begin to ovulate. I will continue to supplement your cortisol supply throughout your pregnancy, with no risk to your baby.

Polycystic Ovaries

Polycystic ovaries occur in 4 percent of women. Women having polycystic ovaries are frequently obese, have few if any menstrual periods, and have abnormal hair growth, which increases with the passage of time. Polycystic ovaries are frequently associated with:

- Ovarian or adrenal dysfunction
- Ovarian or adrenal tumors
- Adrenal hyperplasia
- Cushing's disease
- Hyperprolactinemia
- Thyroid disorders

Although many different conditions may cause polycystic ovaries, the basic mechanism for excess androgen production appears to be the same. The theca cells in the ovary make androgen. (You may want to refer to the illustrations of the female reproductive tract and hormone system on pages 108 and 117.) Normally the follicular (granulosa) cells convert this androgen to estrogen. When this chemical process fails, androgens build up, the follicle fails to mature fully, and the immature ovum remains trapped in the ovary. As the next menstrual cycle begins, last month's deteriorated, malfunctioning follicle continues to manufacture androgens. This local supply of male hormone now interferes with new follicular growth.

Month after month follicles form, fail to rupture, and continue producing androgens until the ovary becomes cystic and can no longer function. If I could see these ovaries, they would appear enlarged, smooth, and pearly white: a result of long-term LH stimulation without subsequent ovulation.

When I find your LH level higher than your FSH level, I can be almost certain you have polycystic ovaries. If you are thin, laboratory tests will probably indicate that you also have elevated DHEAS and normal estrogen levels. If you are obese, I will probably find that you have elevated estrogens, because your fat cells are converting your excess DHEAS to estrogen. Thirty to 40 percent of the women with polycystic ovaries will also have elevated prolactin, and many will have abnormally high DHEAS and other androgen levels. If androgen levels are extremely high, I will look for an adrenal or ovarian tumor.

We no longer recommend the wedge resection (removal of part of the ovary) once performed for polycystic ovaries. Although this procedure often temporarily restores fertility by reducing the amount of androgen production, the surgery permanently reduces your fertility potential by removing egg-filled tissues. In addition, there's a significant risk for adhesion formation, which can also impair fertility.

Some researchers are experimenting with lasers, which they use to "shoot" cystic follicles and destroy their androgen-producing capabilities. This surgical procedure may offer some promise in the near future.

As a rule, women with polycystic ovaries will respond to Serophene and other ovulation induction techniques. You may also require Parlodel and/or cortisol to lower prolactin and androgen levels. If you have polycystic ovaries, you have a good chance for pregnancy. I'll discuss more about ovulation induction in chapter 14.

Hypo/hyperthyroidism

Hypo/hyperthyroidism also distorts the hormonal feedback mechanism. Too little thyroid production *(hypo-)* may cause two fertility problems: increased prolactin levels and persistent estrogen stimulation. (See "Hyperprolactinemia" above.) Hypothyroidism slows down your metabolism and causes "old" estrogens to build up in your blood. This persistent estrogen stimulation tricks your hypothalamus into believing that your ovary is producing enough estrogen, so it tells your pituitary to reduce LH and FSH stimulation. When this happens, your follicles fail to mature and your ovaries do not produce enough estrogen to trigger the LH spike necessary for ovulation. A thyroid hormone supplement will lower your prolactin levels and improve your estrogen metabolism. Occasionally thyroid surgery may be necessary.

When your thyroid gland produces too much thyroid hormone (hyperthyroidism), your metabolism increases and prematurely burns up your estrogen supply so you become hypoestrogenic: you don't have enough estrogen. Since the pituitary never senses that your follicle has reached maturity (signaled by elevated estrogen), it does not release the LH spike to trigger ovulation. Oddly enough, taking a thyroid supplement may turn off the overactive thyroid gland and return thyroid hormone levels to normal, so that normal ovulatory cycles resume. Surgery to remove the overactive thyroid gland is sometimes necessary.

Obesity

Obesity can also lead to persistent estrogen stimulation. The large number of fat cells in women weighing over two hundred pounds manufacture enough estrogen to interfere with the ovary-pituitary feedback system. The elevated estrogen tells the hypothalamus and pituitary to stop stimulating follicular development. When you reduce your weight through dieting and a moderate exercise program, fertility will resume.

The successful treatment of hormonal feedback problems affecting the hypothalamus and pituitary gland generally results in pregnancy. Sometimes these women may also require ovulation induction techniques, discussed in chapter 14.

Ovarian Abnormalities

Cysts, tumors, infections, and endometriosis can interfere with the delicate hormonal balance of the ovary and depress follicle development. Surgical

Table 12-5
Conditions That Can Interfere with Ovulation and Menstruation

Pregnancy

Hypothalamic Malfunction
Emotional stress (endorphins?)
Amenorrhea athletica (extreme exercise)
Dieting, poor nutrition, weight loss, low body fat
Anorexia
Idiopathic (drugs, toxins, medications?)

Pituitary Gland Malfunction
Hyperprolactinemia
Tumor
Surgery
Trauma
Empty sella syndrome
Sheehan's syndrome
Cushing's disease

Hormonal Feedback Problems Affecting Pituitary Gland
Hepatorenal disease
Adrenal disease
Cushing's syndrome
Congenital adrenal hyperplasia
Polycystic ovary
Hypo/hyperthyroidism
Obesity (excess estrogen)

Ovarian Abnormalities
Ovarian cysts
Endometriosis
Infection
Premature ovarian failure

Incidental Fertility Findings
Asherman's syndrome (adhesions in the uterus)
Cervical stenosis (cervix closed from surgery)

Idiopathic (no identifiable cause)

removal of abnormal tissues (cysts, tumors, and endometriosis) will often restore ovarian function. Although antibiotic therapy will clear up the infections and restore ovulation, I frequently become concerned about the condition of the fallopian tubes following an infection. I'll discuss more about resolving tubal problems in chapter 16.

Premature Ovarian Failure

Premature ovarian failure simply means that the ovaries run out of follicles. For unknown reasons some women go through menopause at an early age. There's evidence that a few of these women may have developed an autoimmune reaction to their own ovarian tissue. When this occurs, antibodies form, attack the ovaries, and destroy vital structures. Most of the time we do not know why the ovaries fail prematurely. We can confirm this diagnosis by finding elevated FSH levels.

Unfortunately, when you run out of eggs, you cannot make a baby. However, there are new technologies that suggest you may be able to nurture and give birth to a baby (a donor embryo) implanted in your womb. I'll talk more about these wondrous possibilities in chapter 21.

For a quick overview of the sources of ovulatory and menstrual problems, you may wish to examine table 12-5.

A Note of Concern

If you have amenorrhea or early menopause, I'd like to caution you that you may be at risk for bone decalcification (osteoporosis). Estrogen is vital for the maintenance of good bone structure. The estrogen-deficient athlete (10 to 50 percent of athletic women), for example, will suffer significant bone deterioration within one to three years. Even if pregnancy is not your goal, you may need to supplement your estrogen supply to prevent fractures and irreversible bone damage. Check with your doctor.

13. Finding Out Why
You Have Never Had a Period

Nothing is quite as distressing as being "different." And not having your first period by the time you are sixteen (primary amenorrhea) falls into this category, especially if you have not developed breasts and pubic hair as your friends have. I'm told that the girls' locker room can be just as intimidating as the boys'.

However, delayed puberty is only one aspect of this menstrual disorder. Many other factors ranging from anatomical abnormalities to genetic defects can prevent the onset of menses.

Categorizing Primary Amenorrhea

It's quite likely that if you have never menstruated, you've already consulted with your physician about which of the four categories of primary amenorrhea you fall into. You may, however, be unaware of some of the new options you may have for bearing your "own" child. The road to your "happy ending" will depend on which of the four categories you fall into:

1. *Women who have a normal uterus and ovaries:* If your reproductive organs are normal, you have a hormonal problem which developed prior to your going through puberty: empty sella syndrome, pituitary tumor, adrenal tumor, polycystic ovarian disease, and so forth. In some rare cases your problem may stem from an anatomical abnormality: you may have been born with an imperforate hymen (closed vagina) or with cervical stenosis (closed cervix). These problems affect about 40 percent of women with primary amenorrhea.
2. *Women who have a normal uterus with nonfunctional ovaries:* You may have a normal uterus, but have ovaries that do not contain any eggs (germinal cells). These problems affect about 30 percent of women with primary amenorrhea.

3. *Women who have a nonfunctional uterus with functional ovaries:* You may have normal ovaries and a nonfunctional uterus. These problems affect about 20 percent of women with primary amenorrhea.
4. *Women who have no uterus and no ovaries:* You may have no ovaries and no uterus. These problems affect about 10 percent of women with primary amenorrhea.

Treatment Options for Women with Primary Amenorrhea

Normal Uterus and Ovaries

If your reproductive organs are normal, but hormonal problems are keeping you from menstruating, the treatments for hormonal imbalances outlined in chapter 12 will probably restore your fertility. Should your hymen or cervix be closed to the outside, a minor surgical procedure will open them to allow menstrual flow.

If you have one of the other three abnormalities, you'll want to consider some very different and exciting options.

Normal Uterus with Nonfunctional Ovaries (No Eggs)

If you have a normal uterus and nonfunctional ovaries, your FSH will be elevated, indicating that your pituitary is working overtime to stimulate follicular development. This may be because you were born without any eggs (Turner's syndrome) or because, due to an enzyme defect, your ovary cannot respond to FSH stimulation (resistant ovary syndrome). I can confirm that you have a normal uterus with an X ray (hysterosalpingogram).

Even though your chance for having a baby seems hopeless, studies indicate that with the proper hormone supplement, you should be able to nurture a donor embryo in your womb.

Joe and Toni H. went to a clinic in California for this procedure. They used Joe's sperm to fertilize an egg in a surrogate mother, who remained anonymous. Before the embryo implanted in the surrogate's womb, the doctor washed it from her uterus and transferred it to Toni's. Joe and Toni were able to share all of the experiences of her pregnancy as well as the birthing experience.

Unfortunately at this time only a few clinics offer embryo transfers. However, that trend should be changing as the procedures are perfected. You may wish to read more about donor embryo transfers in chapter 21.

Nonfunctional Uterus with Functional Ovaries

If you have normally functioning ovaries, you can have your own baby. One particular couple comes to mind: Gary and Bridgette D. Although her ovaries were perfectly normal, Bridgette's uterus had been damaged by in utero DES exposure. After five years of "unexplained infertility," she was desperate. Gary and Bridgette decided to go to Australia, where they could use in vitro techniques to harvest Bridgette's eggs and fertilize them with Gary's sperm. Three living embryos were placed in a surrogate mother's womb. Three weeks after the second try, they received a call telling them that they had made a miracle baby.

With in vitro fertilization techniques a doctor can surgically retrieve (harvest) your eggs, mix them in a petri dish (in vitro) with your husband's sperm, and transfer your living embryo to a surrogate mother's womb for gestation. Nine months later you can take home your own baby for a lifetime of joy.

Although these medical techniques are feasible today, many unanswered legal and ethical questions have been preventing widespread use. I suggest you read chapter 21 for the legal and moral issues associated with embryo transfers and surrogate mothers.

Uterus and Ovaries Absent

If you have no uterus and no ovaries, you have several options for having a child. You cannot have a child genetically related to you, because you have no eggs to pass on your genes. A surrogate mother, however, can offer you the opportunity for having a baby who is genetically related to your husband. Using artificial insemination techniques, your husband can father the child and you can adopt it from the surrogate mother. If you are interested in pursuing this type of arrangement, I suggest you read the information on surrogate mothers in chapter 21.

Another option you may wish to consider is adoption. Once they receive their "chosen" baby, many couples who suffer through years of unsuccessful infertility treatment often wonder why they waited so long before choosing adoption. Adoption can be a very satisfying happy ending.

Most women with primary amenorrhea can be helped. Women with hormonal imbalances can have them corrected; women with eggs and no uterus can "hire" a surrogate womb; women with a womb and no eggs can give birth to a donor embryo; and women with no reproductive organs can consider a surrogate mother relationship. With the aid of "miracle medicine," nearly all of the women with primary amenorrhea can look forward to a happy ending.

14. The Road to Successful Ovulation

In this chapter I'd like to reveal how we use the newest technologies to overcome ovulatory problems. With the use of ultrasound monitoring and "instant" hormone assays, ovulation induction has become a science instead of a shot in the dark as it once was. The medications and monitoring techniques work so well that when you fail to get pregnant, I must suspect some other interfering and perhaps undiagnosed condition.

Individualized treatment is far more effective than a preset regimen. Because of this, it is difficult for me to say, for example, that you will be given a certain dosage for so many months and then double that dosage for a certain number of months and so forth. Your doctor will determine the best course of treatment based on *your unique response to the medication*. I can only share with you what I do, and help you to understand my reasoning. With this knowledge you will be better equipped to understand what your doctor does and to ask questions about your particular situation.

Ovulation Induction: Screening Candidates

Minimum Prerequisites

The minimum prerequisites for ovulation induction therapy are the same as those for fertility. The woman needs one open (patent) fallopian tube and an ovary that is able to produce mature eggs. To ensure the best possible response to the medication, all other fertility problems such as excess prolactin levels, endometriosis, uterine abnormalities, and inadequate sperm should be ruled out.

Progesterone Withdrawal

The progesterone withdrawal test will determine which ovulation induction regimen will work best for you: Serophene (clomiphene citrate), Pergonal (human menopausal gonadotropin), or a relatively new treatment option, GnRH (gonadotropin-releasing hormone). Think for a moment about what the progesterone withdrawal test reveals.

If you menstruate in response to the test, your pituitary is stimulating your ovaries to make some estrogen. In order to do this, both your hypothalamus and pituitary gland must be intact and working—at least to some extent. So by prescribing Serophene I can trick your hypothalamus and pituitary into making more LH and FSH, which will "kick" your ovaries into high gear. About 10 percent of women treated with Serophene will not ovulate. They may respond, however, to a combination of Serophene and Pergonal treatment, which I'll describe later in this chapter.

If progesterone withdrawal does *not* cause you to have a period, I suspect a uterine abnormality or that your hypothalamus and/or pituitary cannot stimulate your ovaries to make estrogen. Once I've eliminated uterine abnormalities as your problem, you become a candidate for hormone replacement therapy with GnRH or Pergonal (LH and FSH). Women with low estrogen production (hypoestrogenic) respond best to Pergonal treatment: about two-thirds of them will conceive. Women with a functional pituitary may respond to GnRH. Initial studies and widespread use in Europe suggest that using GnRH to stimulate a "natural" pituitary hormone release may improve results as well as reduce the number of adverse side effects associated with Serophene and Pergonal—hostile mucus and multiple births, for example. I'll discuss more about this experimental technique later in this chapter.

Clomiphene Citrate Therapy (Serophene/Clomid)

Clomiphene citrate is available in two popular brand-name medications: Serophene and Clomid. For the sake of simplicity, throughout this discussion I'll refer to this medication as Serophene, my drug of choice because it may have less of a tendency to degrade the cervical mucus.

Serophene is indicated for the woman who withdraws to progesterone and thus demonstrates an intact hypothalamus and pituitary gland. Serophene works by stopping up the estrogen receptors on the hypothalamus and thus tricking the hypothalamus into thinking that you don't have enough estrogen. In response, the hypothalamus "beats the drum" harder and your pituitary gland produces more FSH (follicle-stimulating hormone), which initiates follicular growth.

Serophene Treatment Regimen

The exact procedure for Serophene treatment will differ from one couple to another. Kathy and Stephen S. had a bumpy but fairly typical experience.

"Dr. Perloe, before we get started could you tell me exactly how all of this is going to work?" Kathy asked.

"Sure." I handed her the Serophene prescription. "Before you leave I'll give you a progesterone injection to start your period. In a couple of weeks your period should start. On the third day of your cycle I want you to begin taking 50 milligrams of Serophene—that's one pill—each day for five consecutive days. It's important that you start on the third day because if you start too late, say on the fifth or seventh day, the drug might disrupt follicular maturation or 'rescue' smaller follicles, leading to multiple ovulation and perhaps to multiple births."

Kathy tucked the prescription into her purse. "How does Serophene make me ovulate?"

"As your follicles develop, they release estrogen into your bloodstream. Normally this estrogen would tell your hypothalamus to slow down. Serophene, though, is masking the presence of the estrogen. 'Thinking' that your ovary isn't working at peak efficiency, you will continue to stimulate the growth of the follicles in your ovaries. Giving your follicles this extra boost for a few days will help them grow to maturity. When your estrogen level peaks a week or so after you stop taking the Serophene, your pituitary gland should release a large dose of LH to free your egg from the follicle."

"When should we have sex?" she asked.

"You should ovulate around cycle days 16 to 18, which are thirteen to fifteen days after beginning the medication. Be sure to keep your BBT chart so we'll know if you're ovulating. Call me around cycle day 20. If your temperature does not rise, we will increase your dose next month. If it does go up, then we'll want to do an endometrial biopsy right before your next period starts: about twelve days after your temperature rise. The biopsy will tell us if your uterine lining has been readied for implantation."

I showed her to my office door. "Now, don't get discouraged if you don't ovulate the first month. It may take several cycles to find the right dosage for *you*."

"Thank you, Dr. Perloe, I'll call you in a few weeks. Wish us luck."

"You've got it."

About a month later Kathy called to say that the progesterone had brought on her period and she had taken the Serophene, but her BBT chart was still flat. It appeared that she had not ovulated. I asked her to come in for another progesterone shot so we could try again at 100 mg.

"When your next period starts, I want you to increase your dose to two tablets a day."

"Do you think the Serophene is going to work?" Kathy asked.

"Remember, I told you that it may take several cycles to fine-tune your dosage. If the 100-milligram dosage fails, we'll try another 50 milligrams. We'll do this until you have a biphasic BBT and an endometrial biopsy that shows you've ovulated; or until I'm convinced that the Serophene isn't going to work—but from your test results I don't believe that will happen."

A month or so later Kathy called and told me that her BBT chart was still "flatter than a pancake." She seemed a bit discouraged, but I assured her this wasn't unusual. I was a little concerned, however, because if she didn't respond to 150 mg, it was unlikely that Serophene would work. She might have to consider giving up her running, and I knew that would be a disappointment. I recommended that she come in for another progesterone injection to start her period and asked her to stop by my office for a few minutes to talk.

"Kathy, I'd like to monitor you very closely this month because I'm pretty certain you will ovulate this time. I want you to get the Tambrands First Response Ovulation Predictor Test from your drugstore and start testing your urine for LH. This nonprescription test will tell you when you're most fertile and it will confirm that you're having a natural LH spike to release the egg. It costs about twenty-five dollars."

"You think this will be the month I'll get pregnant?"

"Well, I'm not sure we've made that much progress. But anything is possible. I also want to do an ultrasound examination on the twelfth day after your period starts. Ultrasound will let me look at your ovaries to see the size and number of your follicles. That will tell us if the Serophene is doing its job."

Several days after finishing her third round of Serophene, Kathy came for her ultrasound examination. We asked her to drink six glasses of water before her appointment, because with her bladder full, the sensitive instrument would give us a better picture.

I picked up the smooth ultrasound wand (transducer) and placed it firmly against Kathy's abdomen. "Ultrasound works by bouncing sound waves off your internal organs. We use sound waves because they don't expose you to radiation.

"You won't feel a thing except me pushing against your bladder." I centered the probe over her right ovary. "This will produce a TV picture that shows me how many follicles you're developing and what size they are.

"There it is—a follicle 10 millimeters in diameter. Let's try the other side."

I positioned the wand over her left ovary, and to my delight I found a follicle 12 mm in diameter. I pressed the button to photograph the follicle. "Let's repeat the ultrasound in two days and see how the follicle matures."

Two days later Kathy returned and I found an 18 mm and 14 mm follicle. "Kathy, you should be having an LH spike any moment. I want you to call me after you test your urine tomorrow morning. If you've had a spike, we need to schedule a postcoital examination for the day after tomorrow. We need to know whether or not Serophene is adversely affecting the quality of your cervical mucus. If you do not have an LH spike, I want to give you hCG tomorrow afternoon. An hCG injection should make you ovulate."

I hoped she didn't have to call, because a natural LH spike seems to work better than an injection of hCG. But about eleven Saturday morning my answering service paged me with her number. Late that afternoon I met her at my office.

"This medication should free your egg within eighteen to thirty-six hours. If possible, you should have intercourse tomorrow and Monday morning. There's always a chance that you could get pregnant this cycle, although that would be a stroke of extraordinary luck.

"I want to schedule you for a postcoital examination Monday morning so I can check your cervical mucus. I'll need to see you within two to four hours of your having intercourse."

When I did the postcoital examination Monday morning, I found that Kathy's mucus was scant and very thick. I can't say I was too surprised, since nearly half of the women on clomiphene therapy suffer from mucus problems. I gave her a prescription for low-dose estrogen to use from day 8 through day 14 of her next cycle. I hoped that by adding the estrogen we could improve the mucus so Steven's sperm could swim through.

Kathy returned four days later for an ultrasound test to confirm that she'd ovulated. I was happy to report that I saw a large corpus luteum. So I asked her to return around cycle day 26 to do an endometrial biopsy. I wanted to see if her uterine lining had been properly stimulated.

But the biopsy showed that her uterine lining hadn't developed normally. Even if she had conceived, the embryo might not have implanted and developed.

"Don't be discouraged," I told her. "Nearly one-third of all women taking this treatment have a luteal phase defect. I'd like to give you progesterone suppositories next month to see if that will correct the problem. Go ahead and use the First Response test again. I believe we'll still have to give you an hCG injection before you'll ovulate, but there's no sense in giving you the hCG injection if you have an LH spike on your own. We'll repeat the ultrasound just before midcycle because the hCG must be given at exactly the right time or it won't work.

"I believe we have most of your problems under control." I leaned against the counter. "You know, it's discouraging for me, too, when a new problem shows up in each cycle. But if you look at it as tackling one problem at a time, it makes solving your fertility problem manageable. The only thing I'm still concerned about is your mucus. If the estrogen doesn't clear that up next month, you may want to try artificial insemination. Maybe you should talk about it with Steven."

The next month she repeated the procedure: 150 mg of Serophene for five days, low-dose estrogen to thin her mucus, First Response test strips to detect LH, ultrasound examinations until a mature follicle developed, an hCG injection to stimulate ovulation, and a postcoital test.

When I repeated the postcoital test the fourth month, I was disappointed to learn that the estrogen had not improved Kathy's mucus quality. Steven's sperm didn't have a chance to get through. I told her that since the estrogen wasn't working she wouldn't need to use it the next month. I suggested that instead they try intrauterine artificial insemination (IAIH) with Steven's sperm. She said that she and Steven had discussed IAIH and that it was all right with both of them.

I reminded her to insert the progesterone suppositories into her vagina twice a day for fourteen days beginning the second day of her temperature elevation. I wanted to repeat the endometrial biopsy near the end of this cycle to make sure that her uterine lining had been stimulated.

When I did the biopsy this time, I was happy to report that the progesterone suppositories had corrected her luteal phase defect. Kathy had had a normal ovulatory cycle—well, almost normal—for the first time in two years. In the next cycle we'd try IAIH.

The fifth month we began monitoring the development of a 13 mm follicle. When it reached 19 mm, I gave her hCG and told her to bring Steven with her the next day for IAIH.

"Before this is over, you are going to know as much about this process as I do," I laughed. "I want to repeat the IAIH tomorrow so we'll have plenty of Steven's sperm swimming around when your egg comes along."

Both inseminations went well, and her BBT rise confirmed that she had ovulated and that the corpus luteum had formed. Now all we had to do was wait. If her BBT stayed up and her period did not start, we'd know she was pregnant.

I guess it wasn't meant to happen—not that month, anyway. Kathy called a couple of weeks later to tell me that her period had started. "Don't worry," I said. "We've got you on the right routine now and it's only a matter of time. It may take three or four more normal cycles before we make that baby."

Each month I could tell that it was becoming harder for them to keep up their optimism. I assured them that Kathy's cycles were working fine on this regimen and that it was only a matter of time. Three weeks after their third IAIH she called me. "Dr. Perloe, I think we did it. My period is four days late." Sure enough, that month Steven and Kathy started Jamie!

Diagnosing and Treating Trapped Egg Syndrome

Trapped egg syndrome (luteinized unruptured follicle) seems to occur more frequently in women taking fertility drugs and in women who have had pelvic inflammatory disease. When this occurs, the follicular surface fails to dissolve and release the egg, even though it's stimulated by an LH spike. However, the follicle continues to evolve into the corpus luteum as expected.

Trapped egg syndrome is very difficult to detect. All of the routinely performed tests will indicate that you've ovulated. Your BBT will rise, your midluteal phase progesterone will be elevated, and an endometrial biopsy will be normal. So if you do not become pregnant within four or five Serophene-induced ovulatory cycles, I may perform an ultrasound scan prior to ovulation and just after your temperature rise. This noninvasive procedure will allow me to see your ovary, the developing follicle, and the formation of the corpus luteum. The signs of ovulation include:

- Complete disappearance of the follicle
- Loss of the circular shape of the follicle
- Thickening of the follicle wall
- Replacement of the clear, lucent follicle by an irregular spongy area (corpus luteum)
- Fluid behind the uterus

To prevent trapped egg syndrome, some doctors try to further stimulate follicular growth by giving Pergonal (LH plus FSH). Some add Parlodel (bromocriptine) during midcycle to ensure that elevated prolactins are not interfering with ovulation. Others prescribe a midcycle hCG (LH) injection to stimulate ovulation. Ultrasound examination (or if necessary a laparoscopy) will confirm the effectiveness of these approaches.

Treating Clomiphene Resistance: the Pergonal Short Course

If you are developing follicles with Serophene but they are not reaching maturity, supplementing your LH and FSH with Pergonal injections may provide the results you want.

With the Pergonal Short Course you usually take Serophene plus two ampules of Pergonal daily for five days early in the follicular phase. The exact procedures used during this treatment must be individualized according to your response to the Serophene. If, for example, ultrasound indicates that with Serophene alone you develop several follicles, your doctor will have to add Pergonal very gingerly to avoid stimulating multiple follicles. If you are quite resistant to Serophene, however, more Pergonal may be required. Some physicians perfer trying the short course because it has fewer side effects and is more convenient than Pergonal treatment alone (see below). Many studies show that as a rule women who fail to respond to Serophene are poor candidates for Pergonal induction therapy.

Clomiphene Side Effects

The most commonly observed side effect of clomiphene (Serophene, Clomid) therapy is poor cervical mucus. The antiestrogenic effects of the drug can prevent the mucus from thinning out and ferning in up to 50 percent of women. Sometimes estrogen will improve mucus quality. If the postcoital test reveals live motile sperm in the mucus, pregnancy may be possible. However, in these cases I may recommend insemination with the husband's sperm (IAIH), since it works very well.

Ovarian cysts and enlargement occur in about 15 percent of women taking clomiphene, but complications from them are rare. Small percentages of women report hot flashes, abdominal bloating, nausea, breast soreness, and visual blurring. In addition, I may hear a few complaints about headaches, weight gain, fatigue, and nervous tension. Sometimes it's difficult to say whether these symptoms are due to the drug itself or to the stress of ovulation induction therapy.

Clomiphene does not increase the odds that you'll have an early pregnancy loss or that your baby will have birth defects. The rates of abortion, multiple pregnancies, and congenital abnormalities are all within normal limits.

Success Rates with Clomiphene

Of the women who withdraw to progesterone, 70 to 90 percent taking clomiphene citrate will ovulate; and 40 to 60 percent will conceive within six to twelve cycles. Taking clomiphene will not make you super-fertile. The conception rate approaches that of normal couples: approximately 20 percent per month. The best response occurs in women between the ages of twenty and thirty-five. When clomiphene therapy fails, other fertility factors should be examined more closely.

Human Gonadotropin Therapy (Pergonal)

Normally the hypothalamus secretes GnRH to stimulate LH and FSH production by the pituitary gland. The gonadotropins (LH and FSH) act on the ovaries to initiate follicular development, estrogen production, and ovulation. Sometimes, however, due to an intrinsic problem with the hypothalamus or pituitary gland, the pituitary cannot produce adequate amounts of these hormones. As a result, the understimulated ovaries fail to produce estrogen and fail to ovulate. Typically these women will not withdraw to progesterone unless an estrogen supplement is used to prime the growth of the uterine lining. If elevated FSH levels indicate ovarian failure, Pergonal will not be successful.

The Pergonal Treatment Regimen

There are many different ways to use Pergonal, but a few standards must be strictly followed. Estrogen assays and ultrasound examinations must be performed regularly in order to avoid multiple births and life-threatening complications. If your doctor prescribes Pergonal without taking these precautions, I suggest you consult with a different physician.

Pergonal treatment can be very demanding and expensive, averaging about $1,000 per treatment cycle. The woman must come to the doctor's office for daily injections, for periodic blood tests, and for ultrasound evaluations. You and your spouse must be prepared for the rigors of this schedule or you won't make it.

I'd like to share with you the experience Tammy and Ken J. had with Pergonal treatments. They had really been through the wringer. After five disappointing years I was the third doctor they had consulted. Tammy had received Pergonal before, but her doctor had not used ultrasound to monitor follicular development. Since we started using ultrasound, pregnancy rates with Pergonal therapy have doubled. So I recommended that they give it another try.

Before starting their treatment I ordered a blood test to measure Tammy's normal estrogen level. As you'll see, this reference point helped me determine the amount of Pergonal I should give her.

Studies show that a month or two of estrogen pretreatment will improve cervical mucus and the uterine environment. A month before starting Pergonal I gave Tammy estrogen for twenty-five days and progesterone for five days, thereby inducing a "normal" menstrual cycle.

After Tammy's period began, I gave her two ampules of Pergonal (150 units FSH and 150 units LH) for three consecutive days (see figure 14-1). At that time I measured her estrogen once more and compared it to her baseline. If the medication was adequately stimulating follicular growth, her estrogen would double. Since I saw no significant increase in her estrogen, I increased the dosage by 50 percent (to three ampules per day) and repeated the estrogen test in three days. I would repeat this procedure until she achieved an estrogen response indicative of follicular development. Once Tammy's estrogen doubled over a three-day period, I continued giving her that dose of Pergonal.

When Tammy's estrogen increased significantly (this usually occurs between the seventh and tenth day of treatment), I began monitoring follicular growth with an ultrasound examination every two to three days. We all nearly cheered out loud when I found three good-sized follicles. When the dominant follicle reached 14 mm in diameter, I began scanning her daily. At 18 mm I stopped giving her Pergonal. Twenty-four hours later I gave her an hCG injection to stimulate ovulation.

I knew Tammy would ovulate within eighteen to thirty-six hours, so I advised her to have intercourse the next morning. Several hours after intercourse I performed a postcoital examination to make sure her cervical mucus could support the sperm migration. Since Pergonal does not usually degrade the mucus as clomiphene does, I expected to find all was well—and it was.

Three days after Tammy's hCG injection, I repeated the ultrasound to make sure she'd ovulated and to confirm the formation of the corpus luteum. There it was, just as we'd hoped. Four days after the first hCG injection, I gave her a second hCG injection to prevent corpus luteum failure (inadequate luteal phase). (The second injection may be given four to eight days after the first.)

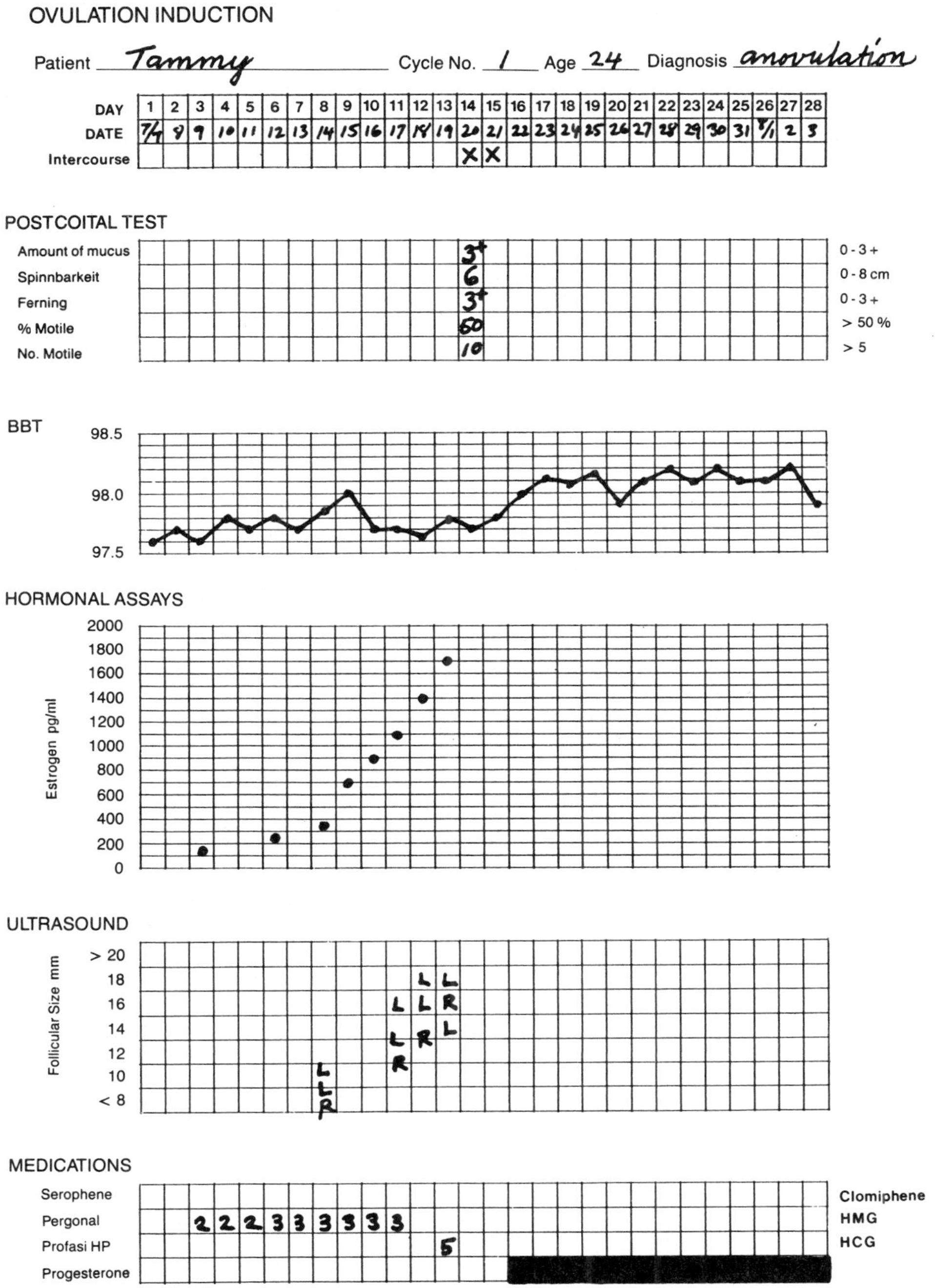

Figure 14-1. Ovulation Induction

Tammy did not conceive in the first cycle, so we tried again when her period started. I began the second round at the same dosage level that produced follicular growth during the first cycle. This cut a week or so off the initial regimen. We all got excited when two follicles reached maturity at the same time. Even though we knew she might have twins (music to her ears), I gave her the hCG injection. Nine months later Tammy and Ken delivered an eight-pound twelve-ounce baby girl.

Side Effects

If estrogen levels become extremely high (over 2,000 picograms per milliliter: 2,000 pg/ml) or if ultrasound reveals numerous large follicles, withholding the hCG injection will prevent life-threatening complications. This mild form of hyperstimulation, which occurs in 10 to 20 percent of all Pergonal treatment cycles, may double ovary size and cause lower abdominal discomfort. After the next menstrual period the swollen ovaries will return to normal proportions on their own.

Moderate hyperstimulation after an hCG injection occurs in 1 to 6 percent of the treatment cycles. With this more serious form of hyperstimulation, the ovaries become cystic and in this fragile condition may hemorrhage, rupture, or twist to cut off their blood supply (torsion). Immediate hospitalization and bed rest will prevent complications. In addition, the patient may need pain medication and intravenous fluids.

Moderate hyperstimulation will usually resolve itself in three to ten days, with complete recovery occurring in four weeks. Unless hemorrhage or torsion is highly suspected, surgery should not be attempted. The ovaries are so fragile during this period that any surgical intervention usually ends with the surgeon having to remove the ovary.

Severe hyperstimulation, a very rare occurrence, causes massive ovarian enlargement, life-threatening fluid/electrolyte shifts, and vascular collapse. Immediate hospitalization and emergency measures must be taken to prevent death. The possibility of this happening is very real for patients who are not closely monitored during Pergonal therapy.

Close monitoring of estrogen levels and regular ultrasound examinations will also help guard against multiple gestations. Each mature follicle contributes 450 to 650 pg/ml of estrogen. During each cycle there may be as many as a dozen follicles growing, with each one contributing some amount to the estrogen pool. Studies show that as long as the total estrogen level is below 2,000 pg/ml the odds of having a "litter" are small. When estrogen rises above 2,000 pg/ml, or multiple follicles are seen on ultrasound, withholding the hCG injection will prevent multiple births and hyperstimulation.

How Well Does Pergonal Work?

Ninety-nine percent of women taking Pergonal will ovulate and two-thirds will conceive. Since the chances for conceiving during any one treatment cycle are 25 percent, most women get pregnant within three treatment cycles. For estrogen-deficient women the pregnancy rate after six cycles exceeds 90 percent. For normal estrogenic women (women who have failed to ovulate with clomiphene) the conception rate is 50 percent after twelve courses of therapy. Women with polycystic ovaries usually respond poorly to Pergonal treatment, generally do better with Serophene, and may possibly do well with GnRH (see below).

Studies show that up to 50 percent of Pergonal patients will get their miracle baby. About one-fourth of these conceptions will be multiple births—three-fourths of which are twins. As encouraging as these reports are, you must also take into consideration that one-third of the Pergonal-induced pregnancies will terminate spontaneously (compared to a 15 to 25 percent abortion rate for women taking Serophene and for women in the normal population).

Women have often thought that Pergonal therapy is a last resort. Now that in vitro fertilization offers additional options, however, Pergonal therapy is far from being the final opportunity for getting your miracle baby. We'll discuss more about that in a later chapter.

Gonadotropic-Releasing Hormone (GnRH)

For years Europeans have been using GnRH to stimulate the pituitary to function normally. Research shows that GnRH therapy seems to avoid the risks associated with hyperstimulation and multiple births. GnRH may also eliminate the need for daily injections and monitoring, and ultimately may reduce treatment costs. So if it's this good, why aren't we using it in the United States? I'll tell you some of the reasons.

Treatment Regimen

GnRH therapy may restore fertility to women who have hypothalamic disorders and an intact pituitary gland. A normal hypothalamus pulses GnRH every ninety minutes to permit pituitary function. So when you supplement GnRH, it must be pulsed in a similar manner. Only recently have relatively inexpensive ($2,000 to $3,000) automatic pumps been developed for intravenous injections: for example, the AutoSyringe infusion pump supplied by Travenol Laboratories and the Pulsamat from Ferring Laboratories. These battery-powered devices are so portable that you can carry your mechanical hypothalamus anywhere you go.

Although some women cannot tolerate the semipermanent intravenous delivery system, most appreciate the relative freedom this treatment option promises: no more daily Pergonal injections and blood tests, no more frequent visits for ultrasound examinations, and no more concern about multiple births and hyperstimulation. After ovulation you discontinue intravenous therapy and receive an hCG injection every three to four days to support the corpus luteum.

Results

Pulsatile intravenous GnRH injection almost always results in ovulation, but the pregnancy rate appears to be only around 25 to 30 percent. Though not quite as impressive as Pergonal results, the added convenience, lower cost, and reduced risks justify further investigation into this experimental procedure. At present the cost for pulsatile GnRH therapy is about the same as for Pergonal treatment. Once we are certain that close monitoring is not necessary, however, this could drop to half—about $500 per month. Some researchers are even suggesting that pulsatile Pergonal may be safer and more effective.

A few years ago women with hypothalamic-pituitary insufficiencies had no hope. Now the wonder drugs Serophene and Pergonal give thousands of women an opportunity to have their miracle babies.

IV. When Sperm Meets Egg

15. Sperm-Mucus Interaction: Is the "Chemistry" Right?

"When my doctor did our postcoital test, she said Larry's sperm were dead," Kelly M. told the RESOLVE group. "She also found some white blood cells. She thought one or both of us might have an infection, so she ordered cultures on my cervical mucus and Larry's semen. She also ran some tests to see if we had sperm antibodies."

"What did she find out?" the RESOLVE leader asked.

"Well, Larry's sperm survived in donor mucus. And donor sperm survived in my mucus."

"Then what was killing Larry's sperm in your mucus?" a woman asked.

"The cultures didn't show infection, so she said it was antibodies," Kelly M. said. "My doctor told me that I was rejecting Larry's sperm just like I might reject a kidney transplant."

"What can you do about it?" her friend asked.

"Several things," Kelly answered. "First, we want to try washing Larry's sperm and using intrauterine insemination. If we can get around my mucus, we may be able to get around the antibody problem."

Kelly and Larry M. belong to a special group of infertile couples whose problem we are just beginning to understand and resolve. I'm very excited about the fertility research taking place in the field of immunology. Antibodies, however, are only one reason why cervical mucus may be hostile to sperm. Other mucus problems may also impair their journey to the egg.

Cervical Mucus: Protector and Pathway

Acting as the gateway between the vagina and the uterus, the cervix secretes a thick, impermeable mucus to plug the canal. Normally this "hostile" mucus protects the woman's reproductive tract from invading organisms and foreign particles. At the time of ovulation, however, the mucus transforms into a "friendly" path through which sperm can travel in safety. Under the influence of estrogen the thick and sticky mucus becomes clear and stringy. Like lanes in an Olympic swimming pool, tiny tubular paths form to guide the sperm toward the uterus.

When the mucus fails to become "friendly," as it does with 5 to 10 percent of all infertile women, the sperm cannot safely begin their journey toward the egg. The hostile mucus, as it is called, will either block the sperm's passage or will damage the sperm so severely that they can no longer function. The aim of fertility treatment is to restore the quality of the mucus so it can:

- Facilitate or interfere with sperm transport at appropriate times of the month
- Protect the sperm from the acidic vaginal environment
- Preserve the sperm in the cervical canal and release them in a steady stream over a period of time
- Filter out abnormal sperm
- Protect the sperm from white blood cells which may destroy them as they would invading microorganisms
- Provide nutrients to the sperm
- Prevent bacterial contamination of the uterus

Performing the Postcoital Test

The postcoital test is the primary tool for diagnosing cervical mucus problems. Performed at the time of ovulation, it assesses mucus quality. When I examine the cervical mucus approximately four hours after intercourse, I look for three things:

- If the husband delivered good quantities of sperm to the cervix
- If the sperm are swimming vigorously through the mucus
- If white blood cells are present, indicating an infection in either partner

If the results of the test are good, I don't worry about the mucus being a fertility problem. If the results are poor, I know that a mucus interaction problem exists or that the test was performed at the wrong time in the cycle (the most common reason for a poor postcoital test).

If on the morning after the postcoital test, the BBT chart does not indicate that you've ovulated, I'll repeat the test every other day until you do ovulate. If your periods are irregular, I can recommend more accurate tests for timing the postcoital test: the Tambrands First Response Ovulation Predictor Test, Ovutime, OvuSTICKS, and/or the CUE Fertility Monitor. (See chapter 14 on ovulation induction and chapter 21 on artificial insemination for descriptions of these tests.) Since we can predict ovulation more accurately than we could when only the BBT chart was available, we are less likely to get poor results from poor timing.

A number of factors can cause an abnormal postcoital test:

- *Infection* in either partner (indicated by white blood cells in the mucus)
- *Sperm antibodies* produced by either partner will cause the sperm to die, to agglutinate (clump together), and/or to shake.
- *Abnormal mucus quality:* High-viscosity and/or low-volume mucus can block sperm.
- *Abnormal semen:* Sperm antibodies produced by the man as well as infections in the man can adversely affect test results, as can a low sperm count and poor motility.
- *Poor coital technique or ejaculation disorders* can also prevent the sperm from reaching the cervix.

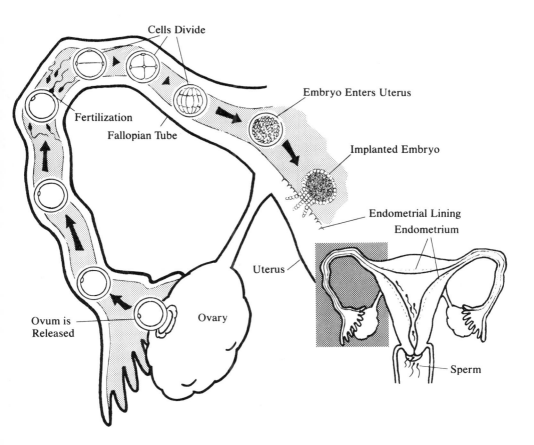

Figure 15-1. When Sperm Meets Egg

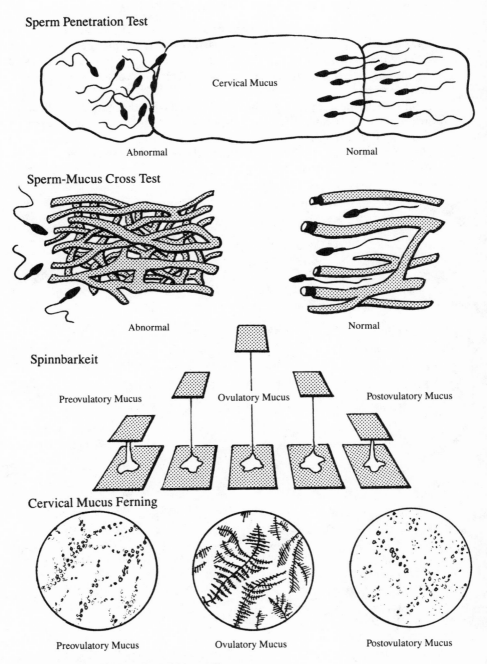

Figure 15-2. Cervical Mucus Test

Infections: Diagnosis and Treatment

Diagnosis
Infectious organisms in either partner may kill or maim sperm. I suspect an infection if I find dead sperm, white blood cells, and/or cellular debris in the postcoital specimen. Specific microorganisms can often be identified by performing a culture of the cervical mucus. In the presence of white blood cells, however, I may prescribe an antibiotic even if the culture comes back negative.

Treatment
Both partners must be treated to ensure that they are not passing the disease back and forth. The semen and mucus cultures for Dan and Marie C., for example, revealed the presence of chlamydia. I prescribed an antibiotic (doxycycline) for both of them. To avoid exposing an early pregnancy to antibiotics, Marie took the medication during the ten days following the start of her menses.

If I continued to find white blood cells in Marie's mucus, I would try to isolate the problem. To make sure Dan was not depositing white blood cells with his sperm, I would ask them to abstain from sex until just before their next postcoital. A normal semen analysis and the presence of the white blood cells *only* immediately following intercourse would tell me Marie was producing them in response to Dan's semen, which could indicate a sperm antibody problem. I was relieved when I found Marie's mucus free of white blood cells after antibiotic therapy.

After the antibiotic arrests an infection, 42 percent of the couples treated will conceive within three months, and 84 percent within one year.

Testing for Sperm Antibodies

The Sperm-Mucus Cross Tests
Normally antibodies attack foreign substances invading your body. For some unknown reason, however, 4 percent of all men produce antibodies against their own sperm. (The incidence of this autoimmunity increases from 4 percent to 50 to 60 percent in men with vasectomies. The sperm antibodies are probably a protective mechanism to help get rid of millions of unused, trapped sperm.) The effects of antisperm antibodies will usually show up in the semen analysis: the sperm may clump together (agglutinate) or shake in random motions.

Sperm antibodies are also found in the cervical mucus of 30 percent of women with unexplained infertility problems. If a fairly recent semen analysis shows that unexposed sperm have normal forward motility, but the postcoital test shows them shaking or clumping, I'll suspect that the woman is the source of the sperm antibodies.

A sperm-mucus cross test will help me understand the exact nature of a couple's sperm antibody problem.

John and Leslie P. were referred to me after four years of unexplained infertility. John's semen analysis was normal and their cultures were negative. When their family doctor did a postcoital, however, he found dead sperm. Since they used the CUE Monitor to predict ovulation, I knew they had timed the test perfectly. The couple obviously had a sperm-mucus interaction problem.

The first thing I did was a cross test. When I put John's sperm in bovine mucus (PeneTrak test), they swam up the tube like little troupers. When I put his sperm in his wife's mucus, they clumped together and shook as if they were freezing to death. When I put donor sperm in a specimen of Leslie's mucus, they looked perfectly all right. Now I knew the problem: Leslie had formed antibodies specific to her husband's sperm.

If I suspect an antibody problem, I also order special tests to look for agglutinating or immobilizing antibodies in the blood, cervical mucus, and seminal plasma.

Treatment for Antisperm Antibodies

Treatment must be focused on the source of the antisperm antibodies. If the woman is producing sperm antibodies, then IAIH, condom therapy, steroid therapy, or in vitro fertilization may help. If the man is producing sperm antibodies, sperm washing with IAIH, steroid therapy, or in vitro fertilization may help.

Intrauterine Insemination (IAIH)

When the sperm from the man are antibody-bound, they can achieve only a 15.3 percent pregnancy rate. Sometimes, though, we can reduce the adverse effects of the antibodies by washing the semen from the sperm and using them for intrauterine insemination. When washing restores function to more than half of the sperm, we can achieve a 66.7 percent pregnancy rate.

IAIH may also be helpful for women producing sperm antibodies. This is what John and Leslie P. decided to try. By washing John's sperm and injecting them directly into Leslie's uterus, we gave his sperm a head start against her hostile mucus. I cautioned them, however, that since Leslie's antibodies could be anywhere in her genital tract, IAIH might not work. Moreover, women with sperm antibodies are twice as likely to have a spontaneous abortion. If IAIH didn't work, they might want to consider AID (artificial insemination with donor sperm).

Although a sensitive pregnancy test showed a pregnancy after the second insemination, Leslie's period started a week later. I was sorry to tell them that she had probably aborted. They were not discouraged; in fact, they were elated. Now they knew that John's sperm could swim to her egg and fertilize it. Undaunted, they continued with IAIH. Two months later Leslie's period was late again. We didn't know whether or not to celebrate because she wasn't out of the woods yet—and wouldn't be for a few months. We all sighed a breath of relief when she entered her second trimester with Mom and baby doing well—Dad, too. Now they have a red-haired, green-eyed baby girl who's made them forget they ever had a fertility problem.

Condom Therapy

Use of condoms during intercourse for a prolonged period of time may reduce the level of the woman's antibodies to the extent that the sperm will not be affected. The woman must avoid all contact with the man's sperm for three to six months; this includes oral sex as well as skin contact. (If the man is producing antibodies to his own sperm, however, condom therapy will not work.) Many people do not want to go this time-consuming route and will elect to use IAIH instead.

High-Dose Steroid Therapy

Experimental therapy with high-dose steroids for men with antisperm antibodies appears to produce a 30 to 40 percent pregnancy rate. Although few studies have been done with women producing sperm antibodies, steroid therapy may prove to be more effective than condom therapy. In addition, suppressing the antibodies may diminish the spontaneous-abortion risk. More research is needed, however, to evaluate this approach fully.

In Vitro Fertilization

By washing antibodies from the sperm and fertilizing the woman's egg outside her body through in vitro, we can avoid exposure to antibodies in the semen and in the mucus. Before attempting in vitro fertilization, a hamster penetration test should be performed on the man's sperm to ensure that once they are treated they will be able to fertilize an egg.

Since sperm antibodies produced by the man or woman are associated with a high spontaneous-abortion rate (50 percent), many couples may wish to try IAIH first. IAIH is much less demanding on the couple and quite a bit less expensive. More research is needed before in vitro can be considered a viable option for resolving sperm antibody problems.

Poor Mucus Quality

Mucus viscosity and volume abnormalities may be caused by surgical procedures performed on the cervix, by in utero DES exposure, and by clomiphene citrate ovulation induction treatment. About 40 percent of the time a low-dose estrogen supplement will improve mucus volume and viscosity. When it does not, or when the estrogen delays ovulation, I will recommend IAIH to bypass the mucus problem.

Women suffering from *cervical stenosis* (scars sealing the cervix) may respond to gradual dilation and estrogen therapy.

Abnormal Semen or Poor Coital Technique

When the semen is poor or when the coital technique does not provide an adequate supply of sperm to the cervix, the postcoital test may appear abnormal, even though neither of these abnormalities represents a sperm-mucus interaction problem. Artificial insemination with the husband's sperm and/or counseling on coital techniques may be helpful in overcoming these problems.

The sperm's journey from your vagina to the egg through your fallopian tube is fraught with peril. Only a hundred or so will survive to encounter this precious genetic package, *provided* your egg can pass into and through your fallopian tube. Unfortunately tubal problems are the most common cause of infertility. In the next chapter you'll learn what can cause tubal problems and what you can do to correct them.

16. Sperm-Egg Transport: Solving Tubal Problems

"I've had abnormal and painful periods ever since I went through puberty," Carrie Y. told the RESOLVE group. "To stop bleeding all of the time, I had to go on the Pill when I was fifteen. The doctor told my mother that I wasn't ovulating and might never conceive.

"I lost my virginity on the operating table. I can't even remember how many D&Cs I had before I was twenty-five."

"Did you cramp a lot?" one member asked.

"Yes, but I thought everyone cramped and that having pain with your periods was normal. The pain eventually got so bad that when I was in my early twenties, I had to stay home during the first two days of my period. I learned later that discomfort from normal periods shouldn't interfere with your daily routines. But since I never knew any differently, all of those years I didn't question it." She paused. "Not until that awful day. My husband and I had decided to try to have a baby. I'd been taking Serophene for several months, to get me to ovulate, and my period was a week late. That wasn't anything unusual, since my periods were frequently forty to fifty days apart. But I'd been regular since I'd been on Serophene. When my basal body temperature stayed up that week, we both became pretty excited. After two years of trying, I was sure I was pregnant.

"But that morning at work I had terrible cramps, like I needed to have a bowel movement. The pain in my side was so bad that I had to go home. Later that afternoon I did go to the bathroom and the pain stopped. But not for long. It became so severe that I thought I was going to pass out. I called the doctor. I cried all the way to the hospital.

"After running some tests, he told me that I had either appendicitis or a tubal pregnancy. I'd begun to spot, so I was afraid I was losing a baby. He had me stay at the hospital overnight.

"The next morning I was weak but I felt better. Since they'd found some blood in my urine, the doctor thought I was passing a kidney stone. And he sent me home.

"The pain continued and the bleeding got worse, so I went back to the hospital and had a D&C. The doctor didn't think I was pregnant because he couldn't find any tissue in the material he removed.

"When I returned home, the pain in my right side was gone, but I was bleeding like a leaky faucet. I knew it wasn't right. I was a D&C expert by then. Another thing that puzzled me was that my breasts were still swollen and tender. But when I called the doctor, he didn't seem very concerned. He just said, 'You can expect some bleeding after a D&C.'

"Even though the bleeding continued, I returned to work. In the middle of the morning, searing pain doubled me over. My secretary rushed me to the hospital. I had an ectopic pregnancy and had lost a quart of blood. That wasn't all I could have lost. I nearly lost my right tube and ovary."

The group was quiet.

"What caused it?" a voice asked from the back row.

"When they did my laparoscopy, they found out that I have endometriosis. That's probably why my periods were screwed up. The doctor said that my adhesions were so thick he could hardly find my tubes."

"What did you do?" a woman asked.

"First of all, I changed doctors. After all I'd been through, I'd lost faith in him. My new doctor is performing a laparotomy next week. He believes he can clean out the adhesions and endometriosis and possibly restore my tubes to normal. He'll also repair the tube where the ectopic pregnancy was. We'll know more after the surgery."

Tubal problems are the leading cause of female fertility problems. With the tremendous increase in PID and sexually transmitted infections, and with the increased incidence of endometriosis, tubal problems account for half of female infertility.

What Causes Tubal Problems?

A number of different problems can impair fallopian tube function:

- Abdominal adhesions and scar tissue that immobilize fallopian tubes
- Adhesions and scar tissue that prevent the egg from entering the tube and traveling toward the uterus
- Damage from an ectopic pregnancy or sterilization surgery

These problems can be caused by a variety of events:

- Ruptured appendix
- Pelvic inflammatory disease (PID)
- Gynecologic surgery

- Postpartum infection
- In utero DES exposure
- Salpingitis isthmica nodosa
- Endometriosis
- Cesarean section
- Bowel surgery
- Ectopic pregnancy
- Tuberculosis (genital)

When infection and disease attack delicate tubal structures, the tubes may become deformed and cease to function. Trapped in adhesions and scar tissue, they can no longer retrieve the egg and coax it toward the uterus. Infection and damage from ectopic pregnancy may strip the vital ciliated lining from the inner walls. When this happens, *sperm cannot meet egg,* and fertilization cannot occur. If the tubes are obstructed only partially, sperm may be able to meet egg, but the developing embryo can become trapped inside the tube and cause a painful and even life-threatening ectopic pregnancy.

The PID epidemic alone is claiming the fertility of hundreds of thousands of women each year. Fortunately microsurgery, laser surgery, and in vitro fertilization techniques can restore fertility to many of these victims.

Diagnosing and Evaluating Tubal Problems

Normal Tubal Function

The fallopian tube is an active, muscular organ that retrieves the egg from the ovary and coaxes it toward the oncoming sperm. If adhesions restrict the tube's mobility or if infection has stripped the tiny cilia from the tubal lining, the tube cannot perform its vital job. The various tests I use will help me determine if:

- The tubes are open (patent)
- The fimbria are open and free to grasp the ovary
- The tubes are free from adhesions so they can move
- The inner lining of tiny hairs (cilia) is intact

I can evaluate tubal performance by tubal X ray (hysterosalpingogram), laparoscopy (telescopic look into the abdomen), and tuboscopy (telescopic look inside the tubes).

The Outdated Rubin's Test

We no longer can justify performing the Rubin's test used to diagnose tubal problems in years past. Simply blowing pressurized carbon dioxide gas through the cervix and out the tubes to assure an open pathway does not define a tubal problem and it does not provide enough information. Today we use more precise procedures to learn the exact nature of your tubal problem—even to the point of seeing the problem with our own eyes—without having to perform major surgery.

The Tubal X Ray: Hysterosalpingogram (HSG)

When to Perform an HSG
When the woman's complaints or history indicates the possibility of tubal problems, the HSG will give me an excellent first look at the problem. I will order an HSG if she:

- Has a history of repeated vaginal infections
- Suffered from one or more episodes of PID or postpartum infection
- Has unexplained infertility
- Has a history of abdominal surgery or ruptured appendix
- Has had one or more ectopic pregnancies
- Wants a sterilization reversal

Purpose of the HSG
By squirting an opaque dye into your reproductive tract and taking X rays, we can see an outline of the inside of your uterus and tubes. The picture will reveal uterine abnormalities as well as tubal problems such as blockage and dilation (hydrosalpinx). If I'm planning a sterilization reversal, I can also see where the tubes are blocked. The X-ray study will not only help me plan the laparoscopy and possible surgery but also help corroborate my other findings.

Performing the HSG
To ensure that an early pregnancy is not exposed to potentially harmful X-ray dosage, your doctor will perform the HSG a few days after your period stops. Before you have the X ray, you may be premedicated with an anti-inflammatory drug, Anaprox or Motrin, for example, or given a local anesthetic. Your doctor will insert a small tube through the cervical opening. By forcing a syruplike X-ray dye into your uterus, the X ray can take a picture of the outline of your uterine cavity. As the dye travels into your fallopian tubes, it outlines the tiny passages.

Interpreting HSG Findings
If the tubes are not blocked by adhesions or scar tissue, the dye will pour into the abdominal cavity. Demonstrating tubal patency is one good sign; however, it does not guarantee that the tubes can function.

The X-ray pictures also give us a rough estimate of the *quality* of the tubal structure and the status of the tubal lining. If the tube bulges, for example, we

X-Ray Findings

Uterine Abnormalities

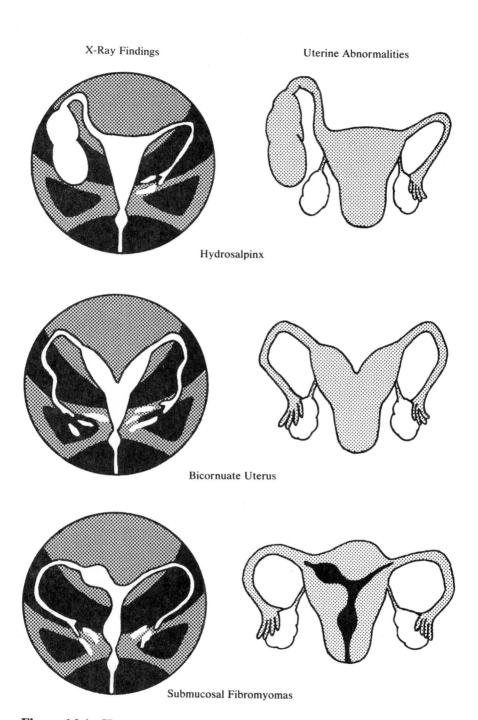

Hydrosalpinx

Bicornuate Uterus

Submucosal Fibromyomas

Figure 16-1. Hysterosalpingogram (HSG)

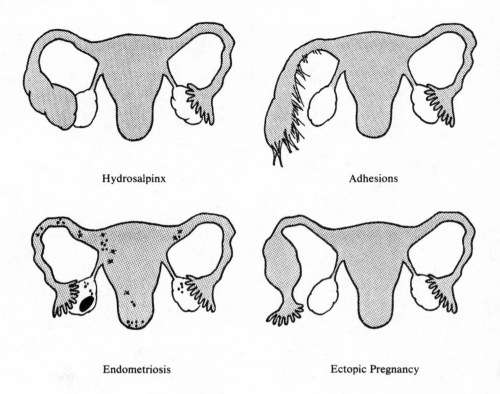

Hydrosalpinx   Adhesions

Endometriosis   Ectopic Pregnancy

Figure 16-2. Tubal Blockage

suspect a hydrosalpinx. And if we do not see the folds inside the tube, we know there are serious abnormalities in the tubal architecture.

We can also see endometrial polyps, submucus fibroids, intrauterine adhesions (synechia), uterine cavity abnormalities, or the aftereffects of genital tuberculosis. Approximately 4 percent of infertile patients will have an abnormal HSG indicating salpingitis isthmica nodosa, a little-understood condition that responds very poorly to surgery. These couples could benefit most from in vitro procedures. The X-ray study may or may not detect pelvic adhesions, mild hydrosalpinx, endometriosis, tubal phimosis (clubbing of the fimbria at the end of the tube), or immobility of the tube.

Therapeutic Effects from the HSG

Although the primary purpose for ordering the HSG is not therapeutic, sometimes forcing the dye through the tubes will dislodge material blocking the tube. Without further treatment a number of women have become pregnant following the HSG.

Potential Complications from the HSG Procedure

Although complications from an HSG are infrequent, there is always the possibility for bleeding, infection, cramping, and the termination of an exposed pregnancy.

Laparoscopy

When to Perform a Laparoscopy

Since the laparoscopy is a surgical procedure done under general anesthesia, I attempt to rule out all other male and female fertility factors before performing it.

Depending on the woman's age and history and the findings from the workup, however, I may choose a more aggressive diagnostic approach for a particular couple. I'm more likely to use the laparoscopy sooner if the woman is in her thirties and/or if I find pelvic pain.

Normally I will perform a laparoscopy for the following reasons:

• Suspected endometriosis
• Abnormal hysterosalpingogram findings
• History of pelvic infection or surgery
• Pre- and postoperative evaluation of tubal surgery
• Failure to conceive after ovulation induction therapy
• Diagnosis of unruptured luteinized follicle
• Diagnosis of ectopic pregnancy

Purpose of the Laparoscopy

The laparoscopy lets me visually inspect your reproductive organs. I can see if the tubes are deformed, swollen, or trapped in adhesions; I can see if the ends of the tubes are open and the fimbria functional; and if adhesions are preventing the egg from migrating from the ovary to the tubes. I can also detect the presence of endometriosis and perform a number of surgical procedures to correct various abnormalities.

Performing the Laparoscopy

If I suspect you have endometriosis, I will perform the laparoscopy shortly after your period stops. Cauterizing the endometrial implants at this time requires less tissue destruction. (See also chapter 17, which discusses endometriosis in detail.)

If I do not suspect endometriosis, I will perform the laparoscopy during the early luteal phase to confirm that you've ovulated. If performed late in the menstrual cycle, the swollen uterine lining may plug the opening to the fallopian tubes and falsely indicate tubal blockage. First, however, I will make sure you are not pregnant by requesting you use barrier contraceptives during that cycle.

A laparoscopy can be performed on an outpatient basis. First, you are given a general anesthesia. Then your doctor will slip the laparoscope through a small incision in your belly button. Through a second puncture just above your pubic bone, your doctor will slip in a small probe to manipulate your organs. Pressurized carbon dioxide gas forces your abdominal wall up and away from the organs so your doctor can get a clear view. After you awake from the anesthesia, you can return home. You may, however, wish to take a day or two off from work following the surgery.

As with the HSG, your doctor will force a dye through your uterus and tubes to demonstrate tubal patency (chromoputerbation). Many times, however, the dye will flow through only one tube (preferential flow) because that tube provides the least resistance. This does not mean that the other tube is blocked; on the other hand, it does not rule out that possibility either.

Many corrective procedures can be performed during a laparoscopy, thus saving the need for major surgery. Electrocautery and laser surgery offer the surgeon safe and effective tools for performing these repairs. Laser equipment and training have been available commercially only since 1984, so we're just beginning to take advantage of all the benefits these technologies provide. The laser is particularly valuable since it limits tissue damage and prevents bleeding, which can lead to further adhesion formation.

The two most common surgical procedures performed with the laparoscope are the cutting and removal (lysis) of thin pelvic adhesions surrounding the ovaries, tubes, and uterus, and the cauterization or surgical removal of endometriosis implants. Sometimes I will sever nerves to the uterus to relieve the pain associated with endometriosis. At present most tubal repairs cannot be performed with the laparoscope, but experimental techniques with the laser offer promise that the laparoscope may be used to release closed fimbria.

Therapeutic Results from the Laparoscopy

About half of the time no evidence of a fertility problem is found. (Oddly enough, of those with no abnormal findings, one-third will get pregnant following the procedure.) Where a problem is identified, about three-fourths of the time it is endometriosis and one-fourth of the time adhesions. If repairs must be made to the fallopian tubes and/or if microsurgery is needed, I will usually perform abdominal surgery. (See the discussion of laparotomy below.)

Once a problem has been corrected (during the laparoscopy or during subsequent abdominal surgery), you will have a 50 percent chance of getting pregnant.

Potential Complications from the Laparoscopy

Although complications are rare, the risks of the procedure include injury to abdominal structures, infection in the bladder or incisions, bleeding,

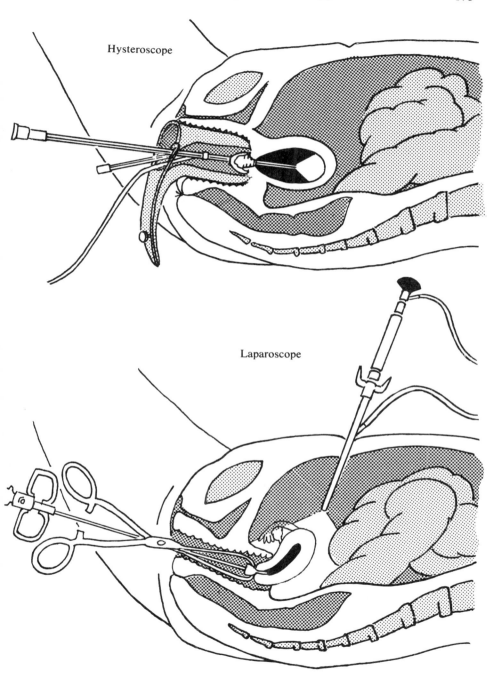

Hysteroscope

Laparoscope

Figure 16-3. Hysteroscopy and Laparoscopy

allergies to medications, complications from general anesthesia, and pelvic infections. Should damage occur to other organs during the procedure, abdominal surgery may be required to correct it.

Tuboscopy

Tuboscopy is an experimental technique that allows us to place a scope directly inside the fallopian tube to examine the quality of the mucosal lining. If I find bare patches, I know that the woman is at increased risk for ectopic pregnancy and that reconstructive tubal surgery will be less likely to restore her fertility.

Unfortunately, at present the procedure requires abdominal surgery to gain access to the fimbriated end of the tube. We hope to perfect the procedure so that it can be done similarly to a laparoscopy. It promises to be a valuable tool for predicting the success of tubal repairs.

Tubal Surgery: the Laparotomy

When to Perform a Laparotomy

I will recommend abdominal surgery (laparotomy) to restore fertility if with the HSG and laparoscopy I discover:

- Thick adhesions freezing the pelvic organs in place
- Organs adhering to one another or to the abdominal wall
- Clubbed (closed) fimbria
- Blocked and/or grossly deformed fallopian tubes (hydrosalpinx)
- Ovarian (chocolate) cysts (endometriosis) that do not respond to Danazol
- Extensive and/or large endometrial implants that cannot be treated laparoscopically

Since the period of greatest fertility immediately follows the first surgery, I may recommend delaying surgery until a time when I have optimized all other fertility factors and the couple is ready to conceive.

Purpose of the Laparotomy

Abdominal surgery affords me the access I need to remove thick adhesions and extensive endometrial implants, to control bleeding, and to repair tubal damage blockage and closed fimbria. I can also perform delicate microscopic surgical procedures with greater safety; for example, freeing ovaries that have adhered to the abdominal wall or bowel and cauterizing microscopic blood vessels. Many of the procedures can be performed with special magnifying glasses (microscopic loupes); some, such as sterilization reversal, require a more powerful microscope.

Procedures Used During the Laparotomy

After you're anesthetized, the surgeon will usually make a bikini cut (side to side above your pubic bone) through your abdominal wall to expose your pelvic organs for inspection and repair. Depending on your fertility problem, a number of corrective procedures may be performed:

Salpingolysis (lysis of adhesions)

In this procedure the surgeon removes adhesions (scar tissue) with a scalpel, electrocautery, or laser. If necessary, the uterus is suspended away from raw surfaces to prevent the re-formation of adhesions.

Salpingostomy/Fimbrioplasty (opening the fimbria and repairing the tube)

Sometimes infection and irritation cause the "petals" of the fimbria to close in on themselves much as a tulip might close at night. Pressure from fluid building up inside the tube causes the tube to dilate (hydrosalpinx). When this happens, it is unlikely that the ciliated inner lining will be intact and functional. I can use a laser or microscopic cautery needle to carve an X-shaped incision at the end of the tube to allow the "petals" to separate and fold back into their normal position. If the fimbria are not restored by this procedure, I can open the tube, but without fimbria the tube has little chance of retrieving the egg. Women with damaged or atrophied fimbria have less than a 10 percent chance for pregnancy. In vitro may offer the best chance for success. (See chapter 21 for a description of in vitro fertilization.)

Tubocornual Anastomosis (removing tubal blockage and reconnecting the tube to the uterus)

When the tubal blockage occurs near the uterus, I can cut out the bad portion of the tube and reconnect the good end to the uterus, with the aid of an operating microscope. I shave away the layers of the uterus over the tubal opening, align the opening with the tube, and suture the end of the tube to the uterus.

Tubouterine Implantation (removing tubal blockage and reconnecting the tube to the uterus)

Another approach for reconnecting the tube to the uterus requires boring a hole into the uterine wall and slipping the tube inside the opening. The tube is then sutured into place.

Tubotubal Anastomosis (removing a diseased portion of the tube and reconnecting the ends; sterilization reversal)

Sometimes repeated infection will block the fluid-filled tube. Removing the blocked portion may restore function to the tube. If it hasn't been stretched too far out of shape, I can remove a section of the tube and reconnect the ends to form a functional passage. The best results occur when the two ends of the tube are similar in size and when the remaining portion exceeds three inches in length. This procedure will restore fertility to half of the women treated.

Sterilization reversals are far more successful than corrective surgery for damage from infection: 60 percent or more will become pregnant after the surgery. This indicates to me that infection often impairs the tubal lining to the point that restoring patency does not restore tubal function. The best success with this procedure has been achieved by surgeons using operating microscopes.

Salpingectomy (removal of the fallopian tube)

Occasionally a tube is in such poor condition that it must be removed or sealed to give preference to the better tube. Bleeding from an ectopic pregnancy may require that I tie off the blood supply to the tube or remove the tube. Provided the woman has one good tube, I may remove a diseased tube if it is painful. If both tubes are not functional or must be removed, I turn my attention to freeing up the ovaries for in vitro egg retrieval procedures.

Removing an Ectopic Pregnancy

If I have any doubt that an ectopic pregnancy exists, I will first perform a laparoscopy to confirm the diagnosis. To remove the pregnancy, however, I must perform abdominal surgery.

Sometimes the pregnancy is small enough that I can simply slit open the tube lengthwise and carefully suction out the material. To repair the tubal incision, I whip sutures around the slit (like whipping stitches around a buttonhole) and the tube will heal normally. Experimental procedures indicate that in the near future this type of surgery may be possible with the laparoscope and the laser rather than through abdominal surgery.

When a more advanced pregnancy ruptures the tube, I will snip out the distorted portion of the tube to remove the pregnancy. Because the tube has a greater tendency to bleed during pregnancy, I will not reconnect the two ends at that time. If within a year the woman does not conceive with the other tube, I may consider further surgery to reconnect the tube.

Removing the Ovary

If at all possible, I try to conserve an ovary. If an ectopic pregnancy implants on the ovary, however, destruction of the ovarian tissue and excessive bleeding may require its removal. The ovary may also have to be removed when it has been replaced with endometriosis (see "Chocolate Cyst" in chapter 17), when it becomes tumorous or when it is painful. Sometimes ovarian enlargement caused by a tumor or cyst may cause the ovary to twist and cut off its blood supply. When this happens, I must remove the ovary. As long as one ovary is intact, however, fertility should not be compromised.

Recovery from the Laparotomy

Recovery should require three to five days in the hospital and four to six weeks of restricted activity:

- No driving for two weeks
- No intercourse for two to four weeks
- No heavy activity or lifting for four to six weeks
- Absence from work for four to six weeks

Potential Complications from the Laparotomy

As with any surgical procedure there is always a slight chance for adverse reactions to the anesthesia and medications; and for postoperative infection.

The Key to Successful Fertility Surgery: Preventing Adhesions from Re-forming

The key to successful fertility surgery is minimizing the damage from infection, from the organs drying out, and from bleeding. Microsurgical techniques cause the least amount of damage, since the specially coated instruments are small and delicate. By using microsurgery we can control bleeding and blood clotting, which may start the formation of new adhesions. We can also use microcautery needles to selectively destroy small areas of tissue—endometrial implants, for example—and to stop the bleeding from very tiny blood vessels. Special solutions are used during surgery to keep the organs from drying out. Before completing the surgery, Hyskon (dextran-70) is placed into the abdomen to restore the slippery, "soapy" quality of the organ surfaces. Anti-inflammatory agents such as Motrin and Anaprox are used postoperatively to help keep adhesions from re-forming.

Follow-up to the Laparotomy

Some physicians will perform a laparoscopy one week after the surgery while the woman is still in the hospital. If filmy adhesions are re-formed, the physician can clean them out at that time.

I often perform an HSG six weeks after the surgery to demonstrate tubal patency. Depending on the nature of the surgery and the woman's age, I may also perform a laparoscopy.

If pregnancy has not occurred within six months to one year, I will repeat the HSG and/or laparoscopy. If I find that the tubes are blocked, there are several different options.

Surgical Procedure	% Pregnancy Rate	% Ectopic Rate
Success Rates from Laparotomy and Tubal Repairs		
Sterilization reversal	60–90	1–2
Ectopic pregnancy tubal repair	40–70	10–15
One good tube and ovary remaining	60	0–11
Salpingolysis	50	10–15
Salpingostomy (90% tubal patency)	33.7	9
Tubal repair leaving less than 3 in.	Poor	
Damage from in utero DES exposure	No surgical correction	

Repeat Tubal Surgery

Tubal surgery costs between $5,000 and $10,000, exposes you to the pain and risks of major abdominal surgery, and may cause you to miss up to six weeks of work. In addition, it may be up to two years before you know if tubal surgery is a success or failure. Experience shows that success rates for repeat tubal surgery are fairly poor. A repeat salpingostomy, for example, has a poorer success rate (less than 10 percent) than in vitro fertilization. The primary difficulty you may have with choosing between tubal surgery and in vitro is that your insurance will pay for tubal surgery, whereas it won't pay for in vitro procedures, which cost up to $5,000 per cycle.

Although in vitro procedures may require traveling to distant clinics and more doctor visits, they expose you to fewer risks than repeat surgery and have a greater chance of success. In addition, within a short time you will know if in vitro will work, whereas with surgery it may take up to two years to find out.

Margaret B.'s Story

Margaret B. suffered a ruptured appendix when she was eighteen years old. She was in the hospital for three weeks and nearly died. At twenty-four she had a PID infection which did not require hospitalization. She'd always been concerned that these infections (peritonitis) could have affected her fertility, but her doctors would never confirm her suspicion.

"At thirty I went off the Pill, and my periods resumed in three months. After six months of trying to get pregnant we became concerned and consulted Dr. Perloe," Margaret said.

"When he did my laparoscopy, he found I had adhesions so thick that he could not see anything else. He told me he would have to do a laparotomy to remove the adhesions and to see what else might need to be repaired. Even though he wasn't optimistic about the results he could achieve with the surgery, we were desperate and wanted to go ahead.

"I was concerned about receiving steroids after the surgery. A friend of mine who'd had tubal surgery a few years ago received steroid injections every four hours. When she came home, she was on a real high, but ten days later she would bawl at the drop of a hat. Dr. Perloe said he doesn't use steroids to prevent adhesions anymore. Instead he bathes the abdominal organs in a solution called Hyskon.

"During my surgery he found that my right tube was blocked and the fimbria had deteriorated. Although he attempted to repair the tube, he was doubtful that it would work. My left tube, however, was in good shape once he removed the pelvic adhesions from around it. After the surgery he told me I had a fifty-fifty chance of getting pregnant.

"After five days in the hospital I returned home. Dr. Perloe told me to stay home; and not to vacuum, pick up grocery sacks, or do any heavy work. After six weeks, he said, I could return to work.

"Three months after my surgery Dr. Perloe repeated my tubal X ray. That's when we got the bad news: *both* of my tubes had blocked up with adhesions. My husband and I didn't want to go through another laparotomy, so we decided to try in vitro.

"I'm happy to report that our second in vitro try was successful! Jon was born last month."

17. Endometriosis: Conquering the Silent Invader

"When we had sex on our wedding night, instead of having an ultimate experience with my husband, sex was so painful I ended up in tears," Marilyn P. told the RESOLVE group. "I thought something was wrong with me . . . that I was frigid or something.

"When I went to the doctor, I told him I'd always had some pain with my periods but that my cramps were getting worse.

"He did a pelvic exam and I screamed when he touched my left ovary. After doing an ultrasound examination, he told me that my left ovary was swollen to twice its normal size. He also felt small bumps behind my uterus. He recommended doing a laparoscopy to find out what was going on.

"That's when I got the news: endometriosis at the ripe old age of twenty-three. What a way to start married life."

Fifteen percent of all women have endometriosis. And with more and more women delaying motherhood until their thirties—the most common age group affected—the disease is having a devastating effect on fertility: over one-half of the women with endometriosis are infertile. For most, once active symptoms develop, the damage may already have been done. And for a third of these women the invasion remains insidiously silent throughout the course of the disease.

What Is Endometriosis and Where Does It Come From?

Endometriosis is a disorder of the reproductive system characterized by endometrial tissue (uterine lining) being located outside the uterus: for example, implanted on the surface of pelvic walls, the fallopian tubes, ovaries, uterus, bladder, and bowel. We do not fully understand how endometriosis gets started. Several theories, however, have been postulated:

- The endometrial tissue migrates from the uterus through the tubes into the pelvis. (This doesn't explain how women with their tubes tied develop the disease.)
- The disease is caused by a genetic birth defect as evidenced by the tendency for it to run in families. Patients with an affected mother or siblings are more likely (61 percent) to have severe endometriosis than those without affected relatives (23 percent).
- Tissue in the abdominal cavity changes into endometrial tissue as a result of repeated inflammation (sheer speculation at this point).
- The endometrial tissue spreads from the uterus to the abdominal cavity through the lymphatic system or bloodstream.

Even a small amount of misplaced endometrial tissue can cause fertility problems. Implants may also rupture during menstruation and migrate to other areas of the abdominal cavity.

How Does Endometriosis Cause Fertility Problems?

Under the influence of cycling female hormones, each month the displaced endometrial tissue grows and sheds blood at the time of menses. Instead of flowing harmlessly outside the body, however, the excrement wreaks havoc in the abdominal cavity.

The resulting chronic tissue inflammation leads to the formation of adhesions and scars, which surround and entrap delicate reproductive organs. The adhesions can be so extensive that they literally freeze the tubes, ovaries, and uterus into place (stages III and IV). The eggs themselves are trapped in the heavy shrouds of scar tissue surrounding the ovaries, and infertility results. As the disease spreads, the older endometrial cells burn out, leaving dead scar tissue in their wake.

Even mild forms of the disease (stages I and II) may interfere with fertility. It is hypothesized that the prostaglandins (hormones) secreted by the active, young endometrial implants may interfere with the reproductive organs by causing muscular contractions or spasms. The tube may be unable to pick up the egg, and the stimulated uterus may reject implantation. Although the mechanism is not fully understood, endometriosis may also result in anovulation (17 percent), cause a luteal phase defect interfering with implantation, or cause a luteinized unruptured follicle.

Some researchers suggest that the woman's body may form antibodies against the misplaced endometrial tissue. The same antibodies may attack the uterine lining and cause the high spontaneous-abortion rate: up to three times the normal rate. (Fortunately, removing the endometriosis with medication or with surgery will reduce this risk to normal.)

The normal tissue surrounding the endometriosis implant becomes puckered and ischemic (suffering from lack of oxygen), causing pain similar to that from a heart attack. Attacked over a prolonged period, the tubes may pucker and swell. Blocked by adhesions, the tubes can no longer provide safe passage for egg, sperm, and embryo. Ectopic pregnancies become a real danger: up to sixteen times more likely than the normal population (16 percent vs. 1 percent).

What Are the Symptoms of Endometriosis?

Nearly one-third of the women having endometriosis have no symptoms other than infertility. The others have varying degrees of symptoms, depending on the stage of the disease. Oddly enough, the early stages or milder forms are frequently more painful than the later stages. We believe this is because the young endometrial tissue liberates spasm-causing prostaglandins, whereas the older endometrial tissue simply burns out and turns into inactive scar tissue.

Table 17-1 gives a profile of the endometriosis patient and tells where the implants, which can be found anywhere in the body, are most frequently located.

Diagnosing Endometriosis

Any complaint related to menses suggests endometriosis. Endometriosis associated with the classic symptoms of painful menstrual periods and/or painful sexual intercourse is relatively easy to diagnose. However, when the symptoms are less suggestive—unexplained infertility, irregular periods, or spotting, for example—identifying the disease may be more difficult. Occasionally while doing the pelvic examination I can feel the telltale beading on the outside of the reproductive organs. The only definitive diagnostic procedure for endometriosis, however, is a direct look inside the abdominal cavity and a biopsy of the tissue.

Laparoscopy

Since laparoscopy requires general anesthesia, I try to rule out all other male and female fertility factors before performing it. Depending on the woman's age, history, and findings from the workup, however, I may choose a more aggressive diagnostic approach for a particular couple. If the woman is in her thirties and if she complains of pelvic pain or has unexplained infertility, I'm likely to perform a laparoscopy sooner.

If I suspect endometriosis, I will perform the laparoscopy at midfollicular phase (around day 7 of the cycle), when buildup and the endometrial implants are smallest. Cauterizing the implants at this time requires less tissue destruction. (See chapter 16 for a complete description of the laparoscopic procedure.)

Table 17-1
Profile of the Endometriosis Patient

(Most common age: 20–35)

Profile of Endometriosis	Incidence (%)
No symptoms	33
Infertility	70
Dyspareunia (painful periods)	28–66
Hypermenorrhea (heavy periods)	12–74
Spontaneous abortion	Up to 50
Weight lower than normal	Up to 50
Weight higher than normal	13
Deep dyspareunia (pain during intercourse)	12–33
Sacral backache (accentuated during menses)	25–31
Pelvic adhesions	24–50
Tender or nodular uterosacral ligaments	34
Uterus tipped anteriorly	20
Anovulation	17
Irregular periods	12
Rectal pain	4
Pregnancy rate (without treatment)	
Mild cases	31–75
Moderate and severe	Very low
Other symptoms	
Inguinal/thigh pain; leg cramps	
Intermenstrual bleeding	
Spontaneous abortion (habitual)	
Premenstrual spotting	

Location of Endometrial Implants

Site	Incidence (%)
Ovaries	61–78
Posterior cul-de-sac (behind uterus)	14–34
Uterine surface	17–55
Intramural sigmoid and rectum	3–4
Cervix, vagina, vulva	Very low

Emotional Side Effects of Endometriosis

Depression
Decreased sex drive because of association with painful sex
Doubts about sexuality
Heightened guilt about sex
Poor self-image

Viewed through the laparoscope, the endometrial lesions look like raised shaggy brown or blue-black areas ranging from 2 to 10 cm (1 to 4 inches) in diameter. If the disease has been present for a prolonged period of time, the tissue adjacent to the implants will pucker and burned-out areas will show fibrotic scars. Advanced endometriosis (stage III or IV) may invade, pucker, and erode the walls of affected organs, and adhesions may be so dense that they "freeze" the pelvic organs into distorted positions.

While performing the laparoscopy, I'll force a colored dye through the cervix, uterus, and tubes to demonstrate tubal patency. Many times, the dye will flow through only one tube (preferential flow) because that tube provides the least resistance to the colored liquid. Although this does not mean that the other tube is blocked, it does not rule out that possibility, either.

Many surgical procedures can be performed during a laparoscopy, thus saving the need for major surgery.

The two most common surgical procedures performed with the laparoscope are the cutting and removal (lysis) of pelvic adhesions surrounding the ovaries, tubes, and uterus, and the cauterization or surgical removal of endometriotic implants. Stages III and IV endometriosis, however, often cause thicker and broader-based adhesions than early endometriosis and often causes the ovary to stick to the pelvic wall. Since the removal of these types of adhesions requires more care than removing the filmy ones associated with earlier stages of the disease, I use laparoscopy to plan conservative surgery (laparotomy).

Since we know that your best chances for pregnancy occur during the six to twelve months following surgery, many physicians feel that more extensive surgical procedures should be postponed to a time when you wish to become pregnant. I'll discuss more about surgical intervention below.

Therapy for Mild Endometriosis (Stages I and II)

Treatments for mild forms of the disease are controversial. Some physicians feel that since adhesions may not form at this stage, it's better to take a wait-and-see approach (*expectant therapy*) rather than prescribing heavy doses of medication. The physician may recommend anti-inflammatory drugs to combat pain during menses. After cauterizing most of the endometrial implants with the laparoscope, up to 75 percent of these women will become pregnant within twelve to eighteen months *without* additional medication. If no pregnancy occurs within six to twelve months, however, another approach may be considered.

Some physicians advise a more aggressive approach if residual implants remain after the surgery. In additional to zapping the implants with electrocautery or a laser, they prescribe suppressant drugs such as Danazol.

Medical Treatment for Endometriosis

Historical Medical Approaches

A number of different types of medical regimens have been tried but discarded because of adverse side effects and questionable results: androgen, estrogen, progestin, and high-dose estrogen-progestin. The aim of all these therapies was to suppress ovulation and menses for a prolonged period of time in hopes that in an unstimulated environment (decidualization) the disease would regress.

"Taking the Pill May Help"

Because many women reported that their symptoms from endometriosis subsided when they were on birth control pills, doctors began using the Pill to control the disease. By suppressing their periods for nine months or more with very high-dose birth control pills, 80 to 90 percent of these women suffered less pain, and nearly half became pregnant when they discontinued the medication. However, endometriosis recurred in a third of these patients. Because of the adverse side effects from high-dose hormones and the marginal results, high-dose birth control pills are not used today to treat endometriosis.

Today's low-dose birth control pill not only may reduce the risk of developing endometriosis, but for many it also seems to provide temporary relief from the symptoms. The Pill may also preserve the woman's fertility by temporarily containing the milder forms of the disease. For these reasons young women with endometriosis may wish to take the Pill until they decide to start their families.

I should caution you, however, that if you suspect you have endometriosis, you should not delay treatment by taking birth control pills until you are thirty years old. By then the disease may already silently have invaded your reproductive organs and made restoring your fertility difficult.

Danazol Therapy

The most popular treatment in use today was introduced in 1975. Danazol inhibits the release of FSH and LH by the pituitary gland. The endometrial implants will improve in 85 to 95 percent of the women taking the drug. Danazol seems to be most effective in women with mild or moderate endometriosis (stages I and II). Menses return four to six weeks after stopping the drug, and the best chances for pregnancy occur about two months after that. Pregnancy rates may be as high as 50 percent with Danazol therapy. Due to the side effects, however, about 5 to 10 percent of the women stop taking Danazol. Table 17-2 illustrates the astounding improvement this drug offers. Potential side effects are profiled in table 17-3.

Table 17-2
Results of Danazol Therapy

Result	Incidence (%)
Pain relief	75–100
Laparoscopic improvement	85–95
Regression of the disease	
75–100 percent regression	33
50 percent regression	50
No improvement	10
Invasive ovarian disease	Very low
Pregnancy rate (up to twenty-four months after discontinuing Danazol)	41–51

Table 17-3
Potential Side Effects of Danazol

Side Effect	Incidence (%)
Weight gain (5 to 15 pounds)	85
Depression	32–62
Unexplained muscle cramps	50–57
Decreased breast size, flushing, sweating	30–56
Mood changes	38–55
Change in appetite	28–54
Fatigue	25–54
Oily skin, acne, abnormal hair growth	25–51
Water retention	28–37
Decreased sex drive	20–35
Increased sex drive	8–35
Insomnia	10–32
Headache	17–31
Nausea	17–28
Deepening voice	7–17
Dizziness and weakness	7–12

Danazol Combined with Surgery

In women with more severe endometriosis (stage III or IV), Danazol may be combined with surgery to provide even better results. Frequently physicians prescribe the medication prior to surgery to reduce the number and size of the lesions. Surgery following Danazol treatment is much less likely to destroy healthy tissue and cause adhesions.

To clear up any remaining endometriosis, Danazol is also prescribed following surgery. Reportedly this approach has nearly doubled the chances for women with severe endometriosis to become pregnant. Some physicians, however, feel that *since the highest levels of fertility immediately follow surgery,* postponing ovulation with postsurgical Danazol treatment may rob you of your best chances for pregnancy.

Buserelin: a Promising Candidate

Experience with Buserelin in Europe may lead to the approval of a new drug which will provide results as good as or better than Danazol and with fewer side effects. Buserelin, or GnRH, comes in the form of a nasal spray. The drug creates the pseudomenopause desirable for reducing the size and number of endometriotic lesions. It is hoped that Buserelin will prove to be a valuable tool in our medical arsenal.

Surgical Treatment for Endometriosis

When Is Surgery Indicated?

The severity of the disease, the woman's history of infertility, the intensity of her desire for pregnancy, and her age all play a role in determining whether or not to do conservative surgery to restore reproductive structures or to perform a hysterectomy.

Mild Endometriosis in Women Under Thirty

If you have been infertile for less than three years and are under thirty years old, I prefer to take a wait-and-see approach. Experience shows that 60 percent of these women will conceive within six months of the laparascopic treatment, without drug therapy. If you are not pregnant within a year or if your symptoms worsen, I may recommend suppression therapy with Danazol.

Mild Endometriosis in Women Over Thirty

If you have been infertile for three years and are over thirty years old, I will begin suppression therapy with Danazol. I may also consider conservative surgery. (See "Laparoscopy" in chapter 16.)

Moderate or Severe Endometriosis and Dense Adhesions

I will recommend surgical intervention to clear adhesions, repair tubal damage, and arrest the progression of the disease. (See "Laparotomy" in chapter 16.) Depending on your age, I may use three to six months of Danazol suppression therapy prior to performing the surgery. Since immediately following the operation you have the best chance for conception, I will often postpone surgery until you are ready to get pregnant.

When Hysterectomy May Be Appropriate

Complete hysterectomy—including removal of the ovaries—is the treatment of choice for women past their reproductive age. With this procedure the recurrence rate is only 1 to 3 percent. Some women with a history of severe pain will request a hysterectomy. After fighting her endometriosis and Michael's retrograde ejaculation for years, Shelley T. decided to have a hysterectomy.

"It felt so good for our fertility nightmare to end," Shelley said. "We could finally have sex for fun. And we didn't have to worry anymore about whether or not my period would start each month. I didn't realize how much pain I had each month until it was over. I wish I'd done it sooner."

Success Rate with Surgery

Where adhesions and tubal damage are not extensive, surgical repairs performed with the laparoscope usually work well. Severe endometriosis, however, will probably require abdominal surgery (laparotomy). The overall pregnancy results from surgery are quite encouraging: 55 to 65 percent. Of those who become pregnant, 30 percent conceived within three months, 50 percent within six months, and 86 percent within fifteen months. Table 17-4 indicates the pregnancy rates following surgery for endometriosis.

Table 17-4
Pregnancies Within 15 Months of Surgery for Endometriosis

Severity of the Disease	% Pregnancy Rate
Mild	70–80
Moderate	55–60
Severe	40–45
Overall	55–65

Using the Laparotomy to Curb Endometriosis

When the adhesions are thick and the tubes damaged, only major surgery will permit the access necessary for performing corrective surgery (laparotomy). You may want to refer to chapter 16 for detailed information on the removal of adhesions and tubal repair.

Since sensory nerves from the uterus run inside the uterosacral ligament, sometimes I will sever the ligament to relieve the pain associated with endometriosis. This often relieves some of the discomfort from labor and delivery, too. To prevent the recurrence of adhesions, I can also suspend the uterus away from raw tissue (surgically treated endometrial sites).

Sometimes the endometriosis invades one or both ovaries and they swell to softball size (chocolate cyst). I can use the laser to slice open the ovary and clean out the debris and old blood. Then I can suture the ovary back together, and the renewed ovarian tissue will once again function normally.

For a complete discussion of the laparotomy and surgical repair of the tubes, refer to chapter 16.

Resolving Multiple Problems Is a Complex Task

Because endometriosis may cause so many fertility problems—anovulation, luteal phase defect, adhesions, tubal blockage, spontaneous abortions, ectopic pregnancies, and idiopathic (unknown) infertility—treating endometriosis can be very complex. I may have to decide if ovulation induction will work in the presence of the disease; or if the endometriosis must be treated before trying ovulation induction therapy. And before even attempting ovulation induction therapy, I must be relatively certain that adhesions will not interfere with fertilization or cause an ectopic pregnancy. If you are at risk for an ectopic pregnancy, medical and laser treatment can reduce your risks for this complication from 16 percent to only four times the normal risk (4.4 percent).

After I perform surgery to remove endometrial implants, clear adhesions, and perform tubal repairs, I must reassess your fertility potential. I need the answers to a number of questions including:

• Are you ovulating?
• Do you have a luteal phase defect?
• Are your tubes open?

Fortunately there are many ways to solve these problems and get all of your systems working in perfect harmony so you will have your chance at making a baby—the greatest miracle of all.

18. The Drama of Life Before Birth: Fertilization and Implantation

How a child arises from the fusing of two cells into one remains one of life's greatest miracles. You've seen how restoring fertility allows the woman's egg to mature, escape from the ovary, and travel through the fallopian tube; how the sperm develop, mature, and swirl by the millions into the woman's vagina. The drama of new life can begin only when all of these events work in perfect unison.

Once the sperm enter the vagina, they must travel to the egg drifting through the fallopian tube. Millions will begin the journey that only hundreds are destined to complete. For every 14 million sperm placed in the vagina, one sperm appears in the fallopian tube within fifteen minutes.

Swimming Isn't the Whole Answer

In the past we thought that the sperm swam the eight inches to the egg. Now, however, we know that even the healthiest sperm cannot accomplish this feat. Researchers speculate that sperm reach the fallopian tubes in two stages. During the first, "rapid phase," contractions of the woman's reproductive tract force the sperm through the uterus and into the tubes. During the sustained phase that follows the sperm use their own swimming power to ascend continuously from the cervical mucus.

They have only a twelve-hour "window" within which to reach the egg. Coursing through the woman's body, the sperm undergo a chemical process called capacitation. Having completed the acrosin reaction, they are now ready to dig through the egg's coatings and fuse with the inner membrane.

We can test the ability of the sperm to fertilize an egg with the hamster penetration assay and the acrosin test.

The Hamster Penetration Test

We can predict fertilization potential by exposing hamster eggs stripped of their outer layers (zona-free) to human sperm.

Collected after seventy-two hours of abstinence, the sperm must be washed free of the seminal plasma within thirty minutes. After a period of incubation they are placed with the hamster eggs for up to eighteen hours. Hamster eggs will allow many capacitated sperm to enter the cell. Within two to three hours healthy sperm should begin to penetrate the eggs. (Due to poor standardization among laboratories, the *number* of eggs penetrated may vary.) Research indicates that bathing the sperm in a special solution may improve their ability to penetrate the egg. However, even if only one sperm penetrates a hamster egg, it proves that the man's sperm can successfully penetrate and that there is a chance for the couple to have a pregnancy.

The Acrosin Test

The acrosin test may provide more information than the hamster test in that it measures the enzyme activity necessary for penetrating the zona pellucida (outer layer of an egg). Early studies seem to indicate a high correlation between the acrosin test and the hamster penetration test. Yet the acrosin test is not only much less expensive but also gives more consistent results than the hamster penetration test.

The Final Courtship

When the sperm locate the egg hidden in the folds of the fallopian tube, they surround it like bees crowding to nectar. In the frenzy that follows, the sperm strip away the cells surrounding the egg, bind to the zona pellucida, and penetrate the perivitelline space below. Then in one miraculous moment a single sperm fuses with the vitelline membrane and triggers a series of spectacular cellular changes which block the entry of all other suitors. That split second seals the genetic fate of the child.

The egg completes its last meiotic division and expels the second polar body, thus forming a nucleus of twenty-three chromosomes to match those brought by the sperm. When the nuclei of sperm and egg combine, and the chromosomes align themselves with their mates, the egg divides and initiates human life.

As the rapidly dividing embryonic vesicle drifts through the fallopian tube toward the uterus, the cells begin to take on individualized characteristics, to perform different tasks. Fluids inside the tube bathe the cells with nutrients and oxygen as the mysterious genetic code orchestrates embryonic development. About eighty hours after fertilization, the cellular mass emerges into the uterus, looking for a new home.

Leaping the Last Hurdle: Correcting Luteal Phase Defect

In the drama of creation one final hurdle remains before the embryo can thrive: the uterus must prepare a protective cradle to nurture the tiny infant. Nature's ingredient for the transformation of the uterine lining is the hormone progesterone.

Produced after ovulation by the corpus luteum, progesterone stimulates the development of the uterine lining so that *at just the right time* it provides the embryo a thick, lush carpet of nutrients. If the stimulation lags only two days behind schedule (luteal phase defect), the embryo may fail to implant in the uterine wall and/or fail to thrive.

Luteal phase defect (LPD) is found in 3 to 5 percent of infertile women and accounts for one-third of recurrent early abortions. Some women with undiagnosed LPD do successfully carry pregnancies, but for those who experience implantation problems or repeated spontaneous abortions, correcting the luteal phase defect is the final step toward ensuring a successful pregnancy.

Diagnosing LPD

Since a single progesterone blood level will not predict endometrial development, using progesterone levels to predict endometrial development requires taking multiple samples. The endometrial biopsy, performed one to three days before the onset of menses, provides the best evidence of uterine lining quality.

Ovulation Induction Therapy and LPD

LPD occurs in one-third to one-half of the women undergoing ovulation induction therapy. When Kathy S. began to ovulate on Serophene, we were thrilled. The thrill was short-lived, however, when we got the result of her endometrial biopsy:

"Kathy, I'm afraid we got some bad news from your biopsy."

"What's that, Dr. Perloe?"

"Your uterine lining wasn't properly prepared for pregnancy."

"What do you mean?"

"Well, there are several possibilities: your follicle may not have developed normally, your corpus luteum may not have functioned properly, or your uterine lining may not be responding to the progesterone. But the effect is the same: your uterine lining won't support implantation. Even if you were to conceive, you might not be able to carry the pregnancy for more than a couple of months."

Kathy looked disappointed. "What can we do?"

"Some doctors like to increase the Serophene dosage to see if stimulating follicular development will improve the formation of the corpus luteum and thus increase the amount of progesterone in your system. But increasing the Serophene may cause other problems, like poor mucus quality. Since you are ovulating on this dosage, let's add progesterone suppositories after you ovulate. We'll repeat the biopsy to see if this does the trick."

The progesterone suppositories worked for Kathy and, as you already know, she became pregnant shortly after beginning the progesterone therapy.

Other Tests

I will also order a uterine X ray (hysterosalpingogram) to rule out several other conditions that could interfere with implantation:

- Asherman's syndrome—adhesions inside the uterus
- Leiomyomata—fibroid tumors inside the uterus
- Uterine abnormalities—septum and other anomalies such as those caused by in utero DES exposure

Treating the Luteal Phase Defect

hCG Injections

Especially in conjunction with ovulation induction and in vitro programs, some physicians will use hCG injections to support corpus luteum formation after ovulation. Studies show, however, that progesterone administration may be more effective in maintaining the pregnancy.

Pergonal Treatment

Some physicians will recommend Pergonal injections to stimulate the development of the follicle during the first half of the cycle. If, however, midcycle ultrasound examination reveals the presence of mature follicles (18 mm or over), the advantage of prescribing Pergonal may be questionable. When the follicles are not developing to maturity, studies suggest that Pergonal treatment will result in pregnancies for one-third of these women. Pergonal results, however, do not compare favorably with clomiphene citrate (Serophene) or progesterone therapy.

Clomiphene Citrate Treatment (Serophene)

If inadequate follicular development caused the LPD, Serophene may correct the progesterone deficiency. Studies indicate that clomiphene citrate will result in pregnancies for 45 percent of women using this treatment.

Bromocriptine Treatment

Women with hyperprolactinemia may also suffer from a luteal phase defect. If tests indicate that prolactin is suppressing progesterone production, taking bromocriptine will usually correct the LPD.

Progesterone Treatment

When ultrasound examination indicates that the follicles are maturing properly, I prefer using progesterone suppositories beginning twenty-four to forty-eight hours after ovulation. If pregnancy occurs, I'll have the woman continue taking the suppositories twice a day up to and possibly beyond the eighth week of pregnancy. At this time the placenta produces enough estrogen and progesterone to maintain the pregnancy. Over half of the women using progesterone will become pregnant. If the progesterone does not seem to correct the LPD, I may try using it in conjunction with Serophene.

The Cradle of Life

Once I correct the luteal phase defect, the stage is set for the fertilized egg to implant in the uterine wall.

The sphere of fetal cells may float within the uterus for up to five days. Once the embryo settles onto a fertile site, the outer cells penetrate the uterine lining and the embryo buries itself within the lush, blood-rich tissue. It's now the twenty-first day of the cycle, a week before menses should begin.

The secretions in the uterine wall will not support the embryo for long. Knowing this, the outer layer of embryonic cells devour their way into the mucus membrane, penetrating blood vessels full of oxygen and nourishment. As these cells multiply, a thick spongy layer of tissue called the placenta begins to develop.

However, grave danger is imminent: the pituitary gland is about to begin its next cycle of activity. If it does, the corpus luteum will deteriorate, the uterine lining will shed, and the tiny infant will wash way. To prevent such a catastrophe, the placenta takes control of the woman's hormonal system and sends out a hormonal message (hCG) which salvages the corpus luteum and quiets the pituitary. The resulting progesterone supply supports the uterine lining while the infant, now only the size of the head of a pin, grows within the uterine wall. After the eighth week the placenta secretes enough estrogen and progesterone to maintain the pregnancy to term, 280 days from the beginning of the last menstrual period.

Menstruation is now one week overdue. The embryonic cells begin to form familiar shapes: a nervous system, a spine with vertebrae, a face, and throat. In the fourth week of its existence a rudimentary heart begins beating. In the middle of the second month of pregnancy the embryo is one-fifth of an inch long and growing about one-quarter of an inch a week. The placenta continues to spread into new territories to provide more oxygen and nourishment.

At eight weeks the baby is no longer an embryo but a fetus; the heart has been beating for a month and the muscles have started their first exercises. Hands and feet experiment with their first gentle kicks. Two and a half months have passed since the last menstrual period.

Twenty weeks into the pregnancy gentle stirrings occur in the lower part of the woman's abdomen, and the rounded stomach begins to protrude. The umbilical cord, consisting of two arteries and a vein, connects the fetus to the placenta, where the mother's blood supply and that of the baby pass only a membrane apart to exchange waste and carbon dioxide for food and oxygen—nature's heart-lung machine.

From the seventh month until term the fetus grows from thirteen to twenty inches and nearly triples its weight. Then one day hormonal messages from the baby signal the end of pregnancy. Uterine contractions become frequent and strong, and the cervical canal dilates so the baby can pass. As the muscular walls compress the uterine cavity, they force the baby down and through the birth canal.

And with one final heave your life changes forever.

19. Death of a Dream: When Pregnancy Doesn't Work

I remember lying there staring into the spotlights. I heard the suction gurgling and instruments tinkling as the doctor flipped them back onto the tray. I knew my baby couldn't survive—not at eighteen weeks. What did I do wrong? Maybe it was the hike we took in the mountains last weekend. Or the long car ride. I can't believe I'm losing our baby. The lights blurred as my eyes filled with tears. I hope it doesn't cry. I don't think I could take it if . . .

"Carolyn? It's all over. You're going to be all right. It wasn't developing normally. It couldn't have survived long after birth anyway. Now you'll be able to have another baby—a normal one. I'll give you something so you can get some rest."

What were they saying? It's deformed? What was wrong? "Where's my baby?" I struggled against the restraints. "Where's my baby?" My eyelids grew heavy as the drug lulled me to sleep. "My baby . . . my baby . . . where's . . ."

Many physicians and hospital workers are not trained to handle situations like Carolyn experienced. They may not know the right thing to say, and when they try to "cheer you up," you may think they're making light of the tragedy you've suffered.

In the past, after a stillbirth, they would quickly wrap the lifeless fetal body and whisk it away to protect the mothers from seeing the horrors of deformity and death. Hospital policies barred grieving mothers from the maternity ward, and doctors quickly discharged them to return to an empty, lifeless house. In the name of expediency the hospital offered to "dispose of the remains."

But what of the *living remains?* What of the exaggerated fantasies parents may have of their baby's deformities? They are lost in expediency—without a baby, without a grave, without a funeral, without the support of family, friends, and a ceremony to help them mourn the death, the loss of their loved one, the missing family member, who will remain faceless and nameless, forever, in the heaviness of their hearts.

Today many medical professionals have a better understanding of the needs of the mother, the father, and the family. We know that the intensity of their grief is unrelated to the length of the baby's life. I treat their loss the same way I would a newborn death. If the parents of a stillborn baby wish, they may hold the infant's remains to say their good-byes. Many people will want to name the baby and make burial arrangements.

With nearly 1 million pregnancy losses occurring each year, you'd think we'd realize that, although it's tragically disappointing to the individuals involved, *miscarriage is a normal phenomenon.* People shouldn't be so quick to blame themselves for doing something wrong, and they shouldn't be so anxious about whether or not it will happen again. Most likely the pregnancy loss was a single incident. *Pregnancy loss does not become a fertility problem until it happens repeatedly.*

Somehow we've grown to expect that every pregnancy will result in the birth of a live, healthy baby. However, this doesn't seem realistic when you consider that 20 to 30 percent of *all* pregnancies—800,000 conceptions each year—end in spontaneous abortion, and over 60,000 babies die after twenty weeks gestation. (I'd like to point out, however, that in the last ten to fifteen years our infant mortality from *all* causes has been cut in half—to about 11 or 12 per 1,000 pregnancies.)

Myths About Miscarriage

Disappointed mothers, fathers, grandparents, and friends can blame miscarriage on almost anything, including jogging, horseback riding, fright, exercise, falling, and even sexual intercourse. But believe me, once the embryo secures itself to the uterine wall, it takes an unbelievably strong force to jar it loose. If a miscarriage occurs after any of these events I mentioned, it probably would have occurred anyway—it was just a coincidence.

When Is Miscarriage a Fertility Problem?

Miscarriages can be divided into two classifications: (1) single, isolated events that will recur only by chance (not a fertility problem) and (2) habitual abortion, where the risk of recurrence is substantially higher than that of the normal population (a fertility problem). The distinction between these two groups is not always perfectly clear. A miscarriage from exposure to toxic chemicals, for example, may be a one-time event if the exposure is temporary, but recurrent if the exposure is long-term.

The following table provides a list of the different factors that can cause either one-time or recurrent miscarriage.

Factors Causing Pregnancy Loss

One-Time Events	Habitual Abortion
Infection, disease, or surgery during the pregnancy	Chronic infection
IUD in place at conception	Uterine abnormalities
Environmental hazards (short-term)	Incompetent cervix
Occupational hazards (short-term)	Environmental hazards (long-term)
Systemic disease (uncontrolled)	Occupational hazards (long-term)
Genetic (isolated accident in fetus)	Systemic disease (chronic)
Severe trauma	Genetic abnormality (inherited from parents)
Hormonal imbalance (temporary)	Immunological (antibodies)
Toxemia	Hormonal imbalance (chronic)
Rh antigen syndrome	Poor sperm
Severe anemia	Increased maternal/paternal age
Umbilical cord accidents	Maternal DES exposure
Premature placental separation	Endometriosis
Placenta previa	Tubal damage (ectopic)
Premature birth (poor care)	Premature birth (recurrent)
Ovulation induction therapy	

Miscarriages before twenty weeks of gestation (spontaneous abortion) almost always occur during the first three months of pregnancy (first trimester). They are most frequently caused by random chromosomal abnormalities or problems with implantation. Later abortions (thirteenth to twentieth week) are usually due to attachment problems with the placenta, uterine structure abnormalities, or a weakened cervix.

If you are in your thirties and have difficulty conceiving, you're at greater risk for spontaneous abortion than younger women who have no difficulty getting pregnant.

Most miscarriages, however, are isolated events that will not recur except by chance. No specialized fertility treatment or expensive diagnostic tests will be necessary to prevent future pregnancy losses. When a temporary condition such as anemia or an active infection is resolved, the risks for having a miscarriage return to normal.

The Warning Signs of Miscarriage

A miscarriage is not a life-threatening situation for the mother. And once it begins, *a doctor can do little to intervene.* To the woman experiencing the miscarriage, however, every spot of blood or cramp may be cause for concern and anxiety.

I remember the first time that I spoke with Nancy V. Before moving to Tulsa she had already had two miscarriages. Now she was in the process of having another. She was frantic. The first day that she began spotting she called me four times.

I asked her to come to my office that afternoon so I could run a few tests. "We'll do a beta hCG today and again in forty-eight hours to see if your pregnancy is developing normally," I told her. "We may need to do an ultrasound to see if the baby's heart is beating."

When I checked Nancy V. that afternoon, I found that she was not bleeding actively and her cervix was closed. We'd have to wait for the second hCG test to find out if her pregnancy was developing normally. Before she left I gave her some instructions:

"You may spot or bleed for as long as a week. Stay off your feet as much as you can. If the pain becomes severe, if you soak more than one pad each hour, or if you get dizzy or light-headed, call me. I may need to do a D&C to prevent complications.

"In two days we'll repeat the hCG test. In the meantime, if you do lose the pregnancy, save any tissue in a clean glass container." If Nancy saved the remains, I'd be able to order a chromosome analysis to check for genetic abnormalities in the fetus.

"Is there anything you can do to save the baby?"

"I'm afraid it is out of our hands at this point. If you do lose the pregnancy, though, I want to give you a complete workup. We need to find out what's causing this problem, and if at all possible, correct it before you get pregnant again. It's not reasonable for you to continue to have this problem."

After we talked awhile, Nancy felt better. As it turned out, two days later her hCG level dropped and the ultrasound showed a missed abortion: the fetus had died in her uterus but she had not expelled it. I did a D&C that afternoon.

When I did Nancy's workup, I discovered she had a septum (a wall of tissue) dividing her uterus into two chambers. I explained that by using the hysteroscope to remove the excess tissue through her vagina, I could probably prevent her from having future miscarriages. She was quite relieved to find out that she and her husband could have a baby.

Threatened Abortion

When an abortion threatens, we can detect if the baby is still alive with ultrasound and with a beta hCG blood test. At six to eight weeks ultrasound can detect the presence of the amniotic sac and fetus, and at eight to nine weeks we can see heart activity. In a normally progressing pregnancy, beta hCG levels should increase 60 percent every forty-eight to seventy-two hours. If the hormone levels are low or do not rise, we suspect an abnormal pregnancy or a missed abortion.

Missed and Incomplete Abortions

A missed abortion occurs when the fetus dies in your uterus but you have little or no bleeding or cramping. You may suspect you've had a "silent" pregnancy loss if urinary frequency and the other signs of your pregnancy disappear—tender breasts, nausea, and fatigue. If you do not spontaneously abort when this happens, you will need a D&C to prevent further complications.

With a complete abortion everything passes out—the fetus and the placenta. With an incomplete abortion some tissue remains in the uterus and may lead to infection and continued bleeding. To prevent your having a septic abortion, your doctor will perform a D&C within a few hours of an incomplete abortion.

When Pregnancy Loss Becomes a Fertility Problem: Habitual Abortion

One or two early miscarriages do not indicate that you have a fertility problem. After one loss the odds of having a miscarriage during the next pregnancy are still only 20 to 30 percent—that of the normal population. After the second loss, however, your odds for having an abortion increase to 38 percent. After the third loss the odds may be even higher.

Habitual abortion—a rather unfortunate term—refers to a woman who has had three or more miscarriages. I say it's an unfortunate term because "habitual" implies she's simply in the *habit* of aborting babies. Nothing could be further from the truth, since this woman has often suffered excruciating losses and, though she wants a baby very badly, may even fear getting pregnant.

When should you become concerned? If you've already had one normal pregnancy, having two consecutive pregnancy losses may be pure coincidence. If you've given birth to an abnormal baby, however, or if you have a family history of pregnancy loss, even one loss may spell trouble. Each situation must be evaluated individually.

Unless my suspicions are aroused by the family history or by a medical history including Asherman's syndrome or in utero DES exposure, I usually won't recommend a medical workup until after the second or third spontaneous abortion. I'll temper my decision by the woman's age and by the couple's level of anxiety about the miscarriage(s). I will also consider a number of other factors linked to recurrent pregnancy loss:

Environmental Factors

A number of adverse environmental factors may contribute to early pregnancy loss. Smoking is associated with a 25 percent greater risk of aborting and with low birth weights. The nicotine from the burning tobacco may constrict the placental blood vessels, and carbon monoxide gas impairs the oxygen-carrying capabilities of the blood, causing oxygen deprivation to the fetus.

Heavy alcohol consumption has been associated with a higher rate of birth defects and brain damage. A number of drugs, including hormones, antibiotics, narcotics, and antihypertensives, may interfere with implantation and the embryonic development (embryogenesis). Excessive caffeine intake (more than ten cups of coffee, or 400 mg, per day) taken by either the mother or the father has also been linked to increased pregnancy loss.

Occupational Hazards

Certain occupations expose women to chemicals linked to miscarriage:

- Metallurgy plants: copper, lead, arsenic, cadmium
- Radio/TV manufacturing: solder fumes (lead)
- Chemical laboratories: organic solvents
- Plastic manufacturing: PVC and other compounds
- Hospitals: anesthetic gas (nitrous oxide)
- Sulfur factories: sulfur
- Hairdressers: chemicals used in hair preparations
- Fishing: methyl mercury from fish living in polluted water
- Industry/agriculture: halogenated polycyclic hydrocarbons

If you are concerned about chemicals you handle on a regular basis, write down their names and show them to your doctor.

Ectopic Pregnancies

Because of tubal scarring from endometriosis, infections, or tubal surgery, the fertilized egg may implant near the ovary or inside the fallopian tube and begin to develop. Few ectopic pregnancies proceed past the third month. Thanks to improved early pregnancy detection and surgical techniques, maternal death from the complications of ectopic pregnancy is rare. The risk of recurring ectopic pregnancies is high. (See chapters 16 and 17 for a complete discussion of ectopic pregnancies.)

The Workup

If a woman has had two or three consecutive spontaneous abortions, I will want to determine if they occurred by chance or if some other factor is at work. If the pregnancy terminated during the second trimester, I'll suspect an incompetent (weak) cervix or uterine abnormalities. A pelvic examination and review of the events leading up to the abortion will help confirm this diagnosis.

If I'm not convinced that an incompetent cervix is the source of the problem, I'll order a uterine X ray (hysterosalpingogram) to study the shape of the endometrial cavity and to look for fibroids and intrauterine adhesions.

I'll also perform an endometrial biopsy at the end of a menstrual cycle to assess the quality of the implantation site. The biopsy will alert me to inadequate progesterone stimulation. I will check prolactin and thyroid hormone levels, since both of these hormones have been linked to early pregnancy loss. I may also order blood tests to check for various medical disorders linked to miscarriage. Semen and cervical mucus cultures will tell me if infectious organisms may be causing the miscarriage.

Genetic studies (karyotyping) are quite expensive, so I will try to eliminate other fertility factors before ordering them. When I do, I usually request a genetic study of the fetus or of the wasted products of the pregnancy (provided they are available). If the baby had normal chromosomes, the genes of the parents are probably normal as well. If the baby shows a problem, I'll then test the parents to see if the genetic abnormality was an isolated event or was passed on by one or both of the parents.

A thorough fertility workup will reveal the cause of the spontaneous-abortion problem. Table 19-1 indicates how different types of problems increase the risk of early pregnancy loss.

Table 19-1
Problems That Increase
the Risk of Early Pregnancy Loss

Problem	% Pregnancies That Aborted
Normal fertile population	20
Serophene therapy	20
Pergonal therapy	30
Endometriosis	40–60
Tubal disease	25–35
Genetic disorders	30
Uterine abnormalities (see figure 19-1)	25
Septate uterus	90
Bicornuate uterus	?
Fibroid tumors	?
Asherman's syndrome	?
Luteal phase defect/endocrine abnormality	35
Male factor (poor sperm quality)	?
Maternal age over 36	31

Breaking the Spontaneous-Abortion Chain

Quite often we can prevent habitual abortions by addressing the problems causing them: correcting hormonal insufficiencies, repairing uterine abnormalities, removing uterine tumors, treating Asherman's syndrome, securing an incompetent cervix, resolving genetic problems, treating endometriosis, treating chronic infection, and/or managing systemic disease. Below are the most common procedures used to alleviate early pregnancy loss.

Correcting Hormonal Insufficiencies

If during the first trimester the corpus luteum fails to provide enough progesterone to support the uterine lining, the fetus will probably abort. This condition is called luteal phase defect (LPD). An endometrial biopsy will tell me if supplementing your progesterone supply during the first trimester can prevent this type of abortion from recurring. After eight to ten weeks the placenta will usually provide enough progesterone to maintain the pregnancy. We cannot be certain how many women have luteal phase defects, since some will carry normal pregnancies. We believe, however, that of those who have LPD one-third will abort spontaneously. (See chapter 18 for a complete discussion of the treatments available for luteal phase defect.)

Abnormal thyroid hormone levels and elevated prolactin levels may also contribute to miscarriage. Restoring these hormones to normal levels will usually prevent future miscarriages.

Repairing Uterine Abnormalities

Uterine abnormalities occur in 1 out of 600 women and cause 10 to 15 percent of recurrent abortions. A misshaped uterus may not be able to support a pregnancy. The most common abnormalities are the septate uterus (divided into two parts by a wall of tissue), a bicornuate uterus, and a double (didelphic) uterus (see figure 19-1).

If you have a septate uterus, the most common uterine abnormality, you can probably get pregnant without any trouble, but you may lose the pregnancy up to 90 percent of the time. A bicornuate uterus may or may not cause pregnancy loss; however, 20 percent of women having one will experience premature labor, and many will present with a breech birth. Even though a double (didelphic) uterus may increase your risk for premature labor, it rarely contributes to pregnancy loss.

I can diagnose structural abnormalities with X rays (hysterosalpingogram), by looking into the uterus with a hysteroscope, and by laparoscopy. As you'll note in figure 19-1, when outlined by an X ray, the inside of a bicornuate uterus and septate uterus will look the same. A laparoscopy will confirm if the exterior of the uterus is heart-shaped (bicornuate).

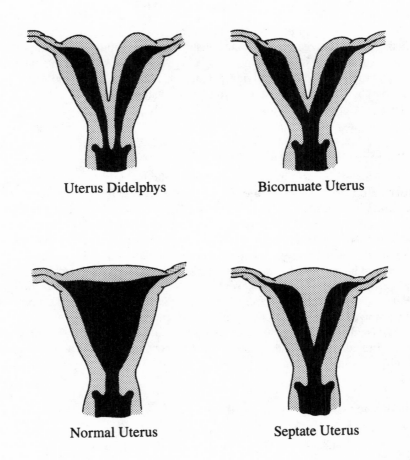

Uterus Didelphys   Bicornuate Uterus

Normal Uterus   Septate Uterus

Figure 19-1. Uterine Structural Abnormalities

When the septate uterus appears to be causing a problem, I can insert a hysteroscope through the cervix and, with some tiny scissors, clip out the excess tissue. An assistant looking at the top of the uterus with a laparoscope ensures that I don't damage the uterine wall. Performed on an outpatient basis, this relatively simple corrective procedure will usually restore fertility to normal levels.

The link between pregnancy loss and the bicornuate uterus is questionable. Unifying the bicornuate uterus requires major abdominal surgery and a cesarean delivery, so usually I will not surgically repair it *unless* it is the only apparent cause for recurring abortions.

Removing Uterine Tumors

Many women have benign tumors such as fibroids (leiomyomata) growing in the uterine wall. Due to a hereditary link, black women are nine times more likely to have fibroids than white women.

Up to half of the women with fibroids will have a history of infertility. We think fibroids may sometimes interfere with implantation of the embryo. If the X ray (hysterosalpingogram) indicates a normal uterine cavity, however, the tumor is probably not causing a fertility problem.

Since major abdominal surgery can cause the formation of adhesions, I do not remove fibroids unless (1) they are the only known cause of the pregnancy losses, (2) they distort over one-half of a uterine wall, or (3) they are larger than 2 cm (1 inch) in diameter.

In the future many of these tumors may be removed through the vagina instead of through an abdominal incision. This experimental procedure is much less debilitating and substantially reduces the risk of causing pelvic adhesions.

Depending on the size, number, and symptoms associated with the fibroid condition, as well as the wish for future fertility, some women will elect to have a hysterectomy.

Surgically removing fibroids (myomectomy) may reduce the abortion rate to normal levels and improve the pregnancy rate to about 50 percent. If the operation does not restore fertility, the fibroids were probably not the source of the problem. If removing numerous tumors weakens the uterine wall, I will recommend a cesarean delivery. Unfortunately fibroid tumors often grow back.

If you have fibroids, you should avoid IUDs, since a distorted uterine cavity has an increased tendency to bleed.

Endometrial polyps occur frequently, but they rarely interfere with fertility. I can detect their presence with a hysteroscopy (telescopic examination of the uterus) and remove them with a laser or by electrocautery.

Treating Asherman's Syndrome

Intrauterine adhesions, usually caused by vigorous curettage after delivery or an abortion, can interfere with implantation of the embryo. Following the D&C you may have a very light period or no periods at all (amenorrhea). A doctor can confirm the diagnosis of Asherman's syndrome with an X ray (hysterosalpingogram) and hysteroscopic examination (looking inside your uterus with a hysteroscope).

I use a hysteroscope and tiny scissors to remove the adhesions. (See figure 16-3.) Following this outpatient procedure, I temporarily place an IUD inside the uterus to keep the walls from adhering. Taking an estrogen supplement for the next sixty days will help restore the uterine lining. Nearly all of these women will begin menstruating, and most will be able to carry a pregnancy to term.

Securing an Incompetent Cervix

I suspect an incompetent (weakened) cervix when a woman has a history of premature deliveries or repeated abortions occurring in the second trimester. Debbie W., for example, presented classic complaints: painless dilation of her cervix followed by spontaneous rupture of her membranes and rapid labor and delivery. An incompetent cervix may be caused by previous surgery performed on the cervix, damage to the cervix occurring during childbirth, and, as in Debbie's case, in utero DES exposure.

At the beginning of Debbie W.'s second trimester, I confirmed that their baby's heart was beating with a stethoscope.

"The heart sounds good and strong," I said. "At sixteen weeks I want to do an alpha-fetoprotein test and an ultrasound examination to make sure your baby is developing normally. Then I'll tighten your cervix with a special stitch that will keep your baby from slipping out before it has a chance to get bigger. You'll be in the hospital for two or three days. Since I'm working so close to the bag of waters, there is always a chance we could disturb the pregnancy. I don't want to take any chances." I set my stethoscope on the counter. "We don't want to lose this one.

"With the surgery you'll have up to an 80 percent chance of delivering a baby. Once I confirm that your baby has matured, I'll remove the stitch. You will probably go into labor and deliver vaginally. If not, I may need to do a cesarean."

As it turned out, the cervical procedure went quite well. When Debbie went into labor six weeks early, we knew the procedure had worked long enough. She delivered a healthy baby girl.

Resolving Genetic Problems

If the tests I perform show abnormal chromosomes (and this occurs in only about 4 to 7 percent of parents), the problem is usually a translocation of genes on the chromosome; for example, a segment belonging to one chromosome may reside on its companion chromosome. Because the two chromosomes *together* contain all the genes the adult needs, the problem may not cause any observable abnormalities in the parent. However, when the mother or father passes along the *single* abnormal chromosome (either the one with extra information or the one with missing information), the baby may be affected. Once this problem is diagnosed, the couple has a one in four chance that their offspring will be adversely affected by the genetic anomaly; and about 15 percent of the affected babies will abort.

Karyotyping both partners will reveal which one is the source of the genetic abnormality. If it's the man, I'll offer artificial insemination with donor sperm (AID) or suggest adoption. In the future I hope to be able to offer embryo transfer to women having this problem. I'll discuss more about this new possibility in chapter 21.

Genetic counseling is providing much needed information to couples with these problems. Knowing the risks, the couple can selectively abort affected fetuses, choose AID, or opt for adoption.

Immunology May Unlock Many Mysteries

Many unexplained pregnancy losses may be linked to unique characteristics of our immune system. Normally the mother's body does not reject the fetus as it would another foreign object, for example, a kidney transplant. However, there's evidence that sometimes the system that protects the fetus may not work properly. When it does not, the mother's immune system attacks the placenta and causes an abortion. Research in immunology promises great hope for providing the answers to these little-understood pregnancy losses. Until we have the answers, AID may provide a solution for these couples.

Sperm antibodies are another little-understood cause of spontaneous abortion. Women with antisperm antibodies (revealed by a postcoital test) will have a 50 percent abortion rate. Sometimes AID can overcome this difficulty. For a full discussion of how sperm antibodies affect fertility, see chapter 15.

The Tragedy of DES Exposure

Women who were exposed to DES in their mother's uterus have an increased incidence of unexplained, repeated early pregnancy losses. Ironically DES was prescribed in the 1950s and 1960s to prevent miscarriage. Later studies proved that the drug was not only ineffective but often caused congenital defects in the mother's offspring. Seventy percent of female babies exposed to DES in utero have a T-shaped endometrial cavity, which may not be able to support a pregnancy. Others suffered cervical malformations (see "Securing an Incompetent Cervix" above) and reduced intrauterine volume. Often a specific reason for infertility or for the high abortion rate cannot be identified or treated.

Treating Endometriosis

Endometriosis may also cause recurrent abortions. Oddly enough, women with severe endometriosis abort less often than women with milder forms of the disease. We believe this is because mild endometriosis gives off potent hormones called prostaglandins which constrict blood vessels and contract smooth muscles, resulting in a greater risk of miscarriage. When the disease advances, the active cells burn out and form scar tissue which does not produce the prostaglandins. So women with severe endometriosis have a near-normal 25 percent spontaneous-abortion rate. For them, getting pregnant is more difficult than staying pregnant. (See chapter 17 for a discussion of endometriosis and its management.)

Treating Active Infections

Ureaplasma is found in the semen and/or cervical mucus of 92 percent of infertile couples, compared with 30 percent of pregnant women. If you have an active ureaplasma infection, you may experience a spontaneous abortion or go into labor prematurely. Although some physicians question the relationship between ureaplasma and infertility, I find that in the presence of unexplained infertility, treating couples for the disease with antibiotic therapy will often result in pregnancy.

Treating Chronic Infection or Inflammation of the Uterus

Asymptomatic ureaplasma infection (mycoplasma) may lead to recurrent pregnancy loss. Chronic infection, including fungal organisms, uncommon bacteria, and genital tuberculosis, may also lead to abnormal bleeding and uterine adhesions. Antibiotic treatment administered to both the husband and the wife frequently resolves these problems. A D&C may be required to clear the adhesions from the uterine cavity.

Managing Systemic Disease

Women with systemic disease may have difficulty getting pregnant, and once they do they have an increased risk for spontaneous abortion. Women with poorly controlled kidney disease will abort if their blood pressure is high or if they are losing an excessive amount of protein in their urine. Women with mild hypertension, however, do not have a higher incidence of abortion. Women with poorly controlled diabetes will abort 25 to 50 percent of the time. Malnutrition, untreated hyperthyroidism, heart conditions, and hepatitis can all cause an abortion. Once these diseases are brought under control, normal fertility may resume.

Stillbirth and Newborn Death

Stillbirth

Stillbirth occurs when the baby dies in the uterus between the twentieth week of gestation and term. Six out of 1,000 babies are stillborn.

The most frequent causes of stillbirths are toxemia, Rh antigen factors, anemia, umbilical cord accidents, separation of the placenta, and infection. Some stillbirths occur from oxygen deprivation during labor and delivery.

Because stillbirth is usually an isolated event, it is not considered to be a significant fertility problem. The only exception to this might be abruptio placenta (premature placental separation) and placenta previa (placental implantation blocking the cervical canal), which may recur.

Newborn Death

Premature birth, which often occurs with multiple births and high-risk teenage pregnancies, is the leading cause of newborn death. These babies live until birth; but the stress of surviving on their own proves too much. If the prematurity is due to genetic problems, uterine abnormalities, Rh sensitization, infection, and so forth, the problem may recur, but the majority of newborn deaths are isolated events.

Death of a Dream

Tony and I sat on the porch swing, staring into space. We were stunned. Our baby was gone; the nursery was quiet, the house was empty. The wind gently rocked the swing to and fro. All our hopes . . . our dreams for a baby were gone. Once again tears rolled down my cheeks. I remembered all of the platitudes:

"At least you didn't get to know it before it died."

"You're young, you can have another baby."

"You need to go back to work and forget it ever happened."

Forget that we lost a child? I looked at Tony sitting next to me on the porch swing, jaw tight, fists clenched. Sensing my gaze, he turned toward me, pulled a tissue from his pocket, and wiped my face. I nestled my head under his chin, and his arms pulled me close. Together we cried.

The Loneliest Grief in the World

Couples who lose an infant have a right to grieve, a right to think of their baby as an individual who cannot be replaced by another baby. Grief for a lost child is the loneliest grief in the world because no one knew your baby—not like you did—safe in your womb, a part of you. It's natural to feel this way.

Grief Has a Face

"I am restless; can't finish anything I start."

"Food doesn't look good. I've lost ten pounds since Allison died."

"We don't want to go out anymore. Besides, it wouldn't seem right—having fun, celebrating. It's so close to the funeral. What would people think?"

"People are so insensitive. They don't understand what I'm going through."

"It's not fair. Teenagers get pregnant every day—and they don't even want to. God must be punishing us."

"It doesn't make any sense . . . none at all."

Men and women experience grief differently and at different rates. The mother tends to grieve longer, cry more, and appear more emotional. The father may bury himself in work or become overprotective. Typically he will resolve his grief more rapidly than she—or will seem to.

The important thing is to try to express your feelings. Show your tears and stop worrying about what other people think. You need to communicate your feelings openly—to your spouse, to your family, to your friends. As a couple you need to take time to understand each other and to share your feelings. And you need to give insensitive people some strong hints on how they can help you through.

Restlessness, guilt, eating problems, depression, sleeping problems, isolation, irritability, numbness, aggression, sexual withdrawal, and jealousy are all normal feelings for grieving parents. You need to accept your humanness, and when you're ready, come to terms with your grief. This is not to say that you should forget it ever happened, but that you should accept your loss and, after a period of mourning, get on with the rest of your life.

I'll discuss more about how to resolve grief, communicate your feelings, and deal with family and friends in chapter 20. Even though at times it may seem hopeless, you *can* regain your happiness. And with medical help there's a good chance you can have a baby you want so much.

V. Awaiting Your Miracle Baby

20. Planning the Rest of Your Life

"It seems like everything is on hold until we get a baby," Margaret B. said.

"We did that, too. We put off buying a house, getting a car, changing jobs, taking a vacation . . ."

"So have we," Bryan W. interrupted. "We spend all our extra money on medical bills. We *can't* do anything else."

"The menstrual cycle takes over your whole life," Steven S. added.

Kathy agreed. "Every time we want to leave for the weekend, I have to go in for ultrasound or Steven has to collect a specimen for AIH. There's no time for making other plans."

"We don't even go to my parents' house anymore," Shelley T. said. "I can't stand all the questions: 'When are you going to give us a grandchild?' Or, 'Why don't you just relax? Let nature take its course.' "

Kathy interrupted. "I don't go to baby showers anymore either. I used to cry for days afterward and I don't need that kind of grief."

"You have the right to avoid painful situations," the RESOLVE leader agreed. "There's no rule that says you have to force yourselves to face these situations all of the time. You have to plan your own life and be true to your own needs.

"You need to give yourselves permission to move on with your lives. Putting off buying new clothes because you may need a maternity wardrobe instead; delaying your vacation because you might miss a call from the adoption agency; keeping your old job because if you get pregnant you don't want to lose your maternity benefits—it can go on and on. Giving up your other dreams and all the fun in your life only adds to your frustration and anger."

Then Margaret B. spoke: "I'm beginning to understand what you're saying. We aren't just upset about our fertility problem; we're also upset about how our fertility problem is ruining the rest of our lives."

"So if we would try to live like normal people, we would be happier."
Richard B. reached for Margaret's hand. "It would do a lot for our marriage,
too."

Even when only one partner must be medically treated, I find that the
fertility problem affects them both because the *couple* loses control of their
destiny, the *couple* undergoes fertility treatment, and the *couple* shares the
emotional strain of dealing with friends and family. Infertility does not just
affect one person; *it affects the couple*.

In this chapter I want to help you rethink the attitudes that may be
interfering with your self-esteem, your sexuality, and your progress toward
pregnancy. You are entitled to have the freedom to be yourself and to
consider new options apart from what others expect or demand. I want to put
you back in control of your life so that you can deal with your marriage, your
family, your friends, and your career. And I'm certain that as a couple you
will grow closer and stronger from your efforts.

Infertility—a Recycling Life Crisis

Coping with a fertility problem is as significant a life crisis as adjusting to
the death of a loved one. Because of the ambiguity of the loss, however,
couples with fertility problems have difficulty getting over their crisis: there is
no body to bury and no clear-cut stopping point. Perhaps it's more like having
a loved one missing in action. There's always hope: just one more month of
treatment, just one more surgery, maybe next month will be The One. With
each attempt the couple develops renewed hope, and with each failure the
couple mourns their loss. Then, once again, they muster up enough strength
to get back on the emotional crisis roller coaster: they try again, and again,
and again.

Riding the Emotional Crisis Roller Coaster

Shock and denial. When you learn that you are "infertile" or that your
fertility treatment has failed, at first you become numb. You may have
difficulty thinking, experience emotional swings and outbursts, and show
impaired judgment. You may only be able to function from day to day and not
really believe the facts: "This can't be happening to me. I'm not infertile, I
just can't get pregnant." "Until now I had a perfectly ordered life; then
everything just hit the wall." This period of adjustment may last several
weeks or even a couple of months

Searching and learning is a period during which you want to learn
everything you can about infertility, so you can make some sense of it. You
read everything you can get your hands on and talk to infertile couples every
chance you get. You may frequently find yourself becoming angry, restless,

impatient, and indecisive. You begin to feel guilty about what you perceive as past transgressions: an abortion you had as a teenager, an affair that caused PID, or using birth control for so many years. During this time, studies show that you are at greatest risk for developing an illness.

Bargaining and guilt is a stage where you attempt to regain control of your life and do a lot of crying. You may look to God for answers or promise to "be good" if you get pregnant. You may find yourself saying, "What did I do to deserve this?" "Maybe I'm too selfish," "It's your fault," or "Maybe we don't deserve children; our marriage isn't the greatest in the world."

Anger grows from the senselessness and futility of the situation. You become resentful, enraged, and feel helpless. You feel that you've lost control of one of your basic rights. You say, "Why me? All sorts of other people can have babies. I'm a good, wholesome person, so why do I have to suffer?"

Optimism and hope grow as you begin to believe that treatment will help. You work hard at your treatment, but your anger and frustration increase with each failure. You may even start to con yourself: "I'm sure everything will work out," "It doesn't really matter anyway," "I should feel happy—I've got everything else I could want," "Maybe if we adopt, I'll get pregnant," "Maybe we shouldn't have any children."

Depression descends from your pain, despair, emptiness, and sadness. For many, life loses its meaning and pregnancy becomes an obsession. You try more bargaining: "We'll do anything." Any failure—at work, at school, in bed—is seen as "another example of my inadequacy." You begin to think that you may be going crazy: "I'm trapped in hope; I don't want to hope anymore."

Reorganization follows depression and is characterized by better judgment, better eating and sleeping. The obsessive drive is gone; you are healthier; you begin to get your priorities into perspective. You stop fighting what's happening and realize that like it or not, fertility problems are part of your life and need to be dealt with, not denied.

Acceptance and resolution take place when the doctor says, "We've done all we can." Once the pain subsides, you begin to say, "Maybe it would be okay to decide not to have children"; "If I never have a baby, I at least have a husband who loves me. We're going through this together and he's right with me"; "I was courageous to get this far." You begin to laugh and make plans to get on with life unless you have renewed hope—a new treatment, a new doctor, a breakthrough in technology—and then you hop aboard the emotional roller coaster for another round.

The time people spend in each stage of emotional crisis varies from one person to another. Their ability to help themselves, to communicate, to handle their thoughts, to manage anger, to adjust to stress, and to resolve conflicts help them move through the stages. People who fail to deal with any one stage of grief get caught—caught in bargaining and guilt, caught in anger, caught in depression. People who learn to deal with each stage, one step at a time, accept their situation, take control of their lives, and start living again. Many of my patients have done this and you can learn to do it, too.

Recognizing the Danger Signs of Excessive Stress

Sometimes stress levels build to unreasonable levels. Your coping skills fail and you begin to use inappropriate and ineffective techniques to resolve your problems. If you find yourself resorting frequently to the mechanisms described below, you may want to seek outside counseling or do some quiet thinking and talking with your spouse or close friend about what is happening.

Displacement—redirecting your feelings from the original person or problem to another person or object. For example, when Michelle P. became upset with her mother, she would take it out on her husband. After her husband gently called this to her attention, they worked out a strategy for her to deal more effectively with her mother.

Dependency—letting someone take care of you and make all of your decisions for you so you are free to "opt out" of life. For example, Vicky M. let her husband take care of all the funeral arrangements for their stillborn child. Vicky always regretted that she hadn't picked out the dress their daughter was buried in. She hated her weakness.

Aggression—moving against another person. Dan M. spent all of his time figuring out how to get back at someone instead of figuring out how to level with the person about how he felt. When he learned to say "Ouch!" he found that people really didn't intend to hurt him, they just didn't understand.

Passivity and evasion—seizing power by becoming passive, by avoiding responsibility, or by pouting. John T. used to say, "I don't care—do what you want," when he really didn't feel that way. Then he learned that people *would* consider his feelings *if he shared them*. That was the first step John took toward taking control of his life.

Sexual withdrawal—expressing disapproval or anger by withholding sexual favors. Not wanting to make love after an argument is understandable, but using sex to get your way is inappropriate.

You may wish to rate yourself on the checklist below. If you have too many pluses for your own comfort, you may want to seek outside counseling. Often a counselor can quickly relieve your anxiety by helping you get your priorities in order and pinpointing the key elements of a problem so you can deal with each stressful situation one step at a time.

Stress Assessment Checklist

Make a copy of this questionnaire or write the statements on a sheet of paper or in a notebook. Then place a plus (+) beside each statement that describes you, a minus (−) beside each statement that does not describe you.

I've lost interest in almost everything but my fertility treatment.

I don't know what to do with my free time.

I spend all day keeping the house spotless/spend long hours on work so I won't think about not having children.

People make too many demands on my time.

I don't seem to be able to say no to my doctor or my spouse.

I don't care what I look like anymore. Sometimes I don't keep my BBT chart or take the medicine my doctor ordered.

I never have any time for *me;* my schedule revolves around my fertility treatment.

Other people's opinions are more important than mine.

I can't concentrate; all I can think about is getting pregnant.

I don't sleep well; wake up too early; don't feel rested. I feel like my body is my enemy.

I nap in the afternoon or fall asleep early in the evening.

I've lost my sense of humor. Without children in my life there's no room for happiness and fun.

I often cry for what seems like no reason.

Sometimes I just feel numb and emotionless, especially about having sex.

Sometimes I laugh nervously and loud.

I want to be alone most of the time. I can't bear having to explain my infertility to anyone anymore.

Life seems superficial. I feel cheated.

I need a lot of reassurance from my friends.

When I'm down, I crave foods, especially carbohydrates.

Sometimes I'm too tense to eat.

I often feel resentful and angry, and don't know why.

Sometimes I wish I could start life over so I could avoid the mistakes that led to my fertility problem.

I often ignore things that in the past would have upset me.

Frequently I'm impatient and irritable. I may even accuse my spouse or doctor of not doing his/her best to help me with my fertility problem.

I think about and talk about the past a lot. Without children I don't have much of a future.

Getting Control of Your Life

Be Your Own Best Friend

Can you look in the mirror, smile, and say, "You are really something special!"? If you cannot, it's probably because you reevaluate yourself every time someone else disapproves of you or something you've done. *Don't let other people knock you off balance* by suggesting a different doctor or a new treatment. Their opinion or point of view is not any more valid than your own. You need to learn to look at yourself, and life, through your *own* eyes. With your experience and knowledge you know far more about fertility treatment than most people. You know where you're going and how you're going to get there. Accept yourself as a "package deal"—overall, you are okay.

Look Ahead

You need to break the habit of living life laced with guilt, always saying things like, "I should have changed doctors two years ago," "If only I had tried to get pregnant ten years ago," or, "What if I had not used an IUD?" Separate your past from your future and move ahead. Allow yourself to change your mind. Give yourself permission to act instead of looking to others for permission and approval. Don't feel as though you have to justify your decisions. Manage your own life. Enjoy yourself and laugh a lot!

Be Assertive, Not Aggressive

Assertiveness is the key to effective communication. By becoming assertive, you can avoid internalizing your anger and frustration. When you communicate your feelings honestly—your disappointment, your pain, your frustration—you help others understand you so they can meet your needs. If they are not concerned about your needs, perhaps you should reconsider the relationship.

You can find out how assertive you are with the following checklist. Try to be as honest with yourself as you can. Your first impression is probably the truest answer.

If your checklist is full of pluses, you don't have a problem with assertiveness. If you have more minuses than you think you should, here are a few suggestions for improving your score:

Plan Some New Responses to Old Problems

Keep track of your assertiveness by reviewing your responses in specific situations. For example, remember the last time someone's insensitivity made you angry? Perhaps someone said something like, "I don't know why

Assertiveness Checklist

Make a copy of this questionnaire or write the statements on a sheet of paper or in a notebook.

Then place a plus (+) beside each statement that describes you; a minus (−) beside each statement that does not describe you.

I usually speak up for what I believe (my doctor, my choice of fertility treatment).

I usually state my views on issues important to me (my right to avoid baby showers, my choice of treatment).

I don't mind complaining openly.

I can say no to my doctor, spouse, and relatives without feeling guilty.

I don't mind disagreeing with the majority.

I don't try to avoid an argument.

I ask questions of my doctor.

I frequently offer suggestions to my doctor.

I can accept a compliment without putting myself down.

I can accept rejection without getting upset.

I can express my anger honestly—especially when a treatment fails to produce a pregnancy.

I can tell someone he/she is bothering me.

I can initiate sex with my partner, even during the infertile days of the month.

I can ask to be caressed.

I can tell my lover what feels good to me.

I can choose not to answer questions about my fertility and plans for a family.

I can ask for favors.

I have confidence in my own judgment about my fertility treatment.

I can let others control the conversation at family gatherings.

I often compliment other people.

I can speak to a group of people.

I can tell my family and friends when I disagree with their suggestions for fertility treatment.

I can introduce myself to strangers.

I can tell jokes.

I do not have difficulty making decisions about my fertility.

having a baby is so important to you. There are other things in the world besides having babies." If you became angry but didn't express it, withdrew from the situation, or found yourself wanting to leave, consider this: Were you upset because of what the other person said or because you were not able to respond? Not willing to stand up for your ideas or your opinions? Many times we are more angry with ourselves for letting others control our emotions than we are because the other person didn't understand us. If you withdraw from the situation instead of asserting yourself, you will probably kick yourself all the way home—and the next day, too.

Imagine handling the situation assertively. What should you have said? Should you have called him a name? Should you have tried to explain your needs? Should you never invite that person to your house again? What are the consequences of these actions? Can you live with them?

If you need some help in deciding what to do, ask someone. Perhaps watching a role model will give you some ideas. Support groups like RE-SOLVE are especially good at showing you how other couples have dealt with stressful situations. Set a realistic goal for the next encounter. Try it out. See what happens. If necessary, modify your approach and try it again. How do you feel? Stick with it.

Keep Communication Open and Honest

Have you ever felt that other people don't understand you, that when you try to talk to them they don't listen? It's hard enough to talk about your fertility problems and the effects they have on your life, let alone trying to get through someone else's thick head at the same time. There are a few principles of good communication which might give you an edge:

- Communicate to be heard, not to win.
- Inform; don't try to teach.
- Make requests, not demands.
- Ask for what you need; don't expect others to read your mind.
- Go for compromise, not perfection.

These principles make a lot of sense, but putting them into practice is another matter altogether. Think about different ways you could say the same thing.

Winning: "I won't go to your sister's baby shower."
Communicating: "When I go to baby showers, I feel awful."

Teaching: "People need funerals to mourn their loss."
Informing: "I really need my family with me right now, to help me say good-bye to our baby."

Demanding: "I need next Wednesday off. I have a doctor's appointment to take some tests."
Requesting: "I need to take some tests at my doctor's next Wednesday. Do you see any problem with my taking a couple of hours off? I can make up the time by coming in early Monday and Tuesday."

Waiting for telepathy: "You know why I'm mad!"

Asking for what you need: "Mom, please don't ask me after every appointment what the doctor said. If anything happens, I'll let you know."

Insisting on perfection: "You ought to understand what I mean! After all, you're a college graduate!"

Going for the compromise: "Would you try to understand? I think it would help us get along better."

I know some of these statements sound familiar to you. As I was writing them, I recalled a few situations I could have handled better, too. Try to remember that you and your mate are a team; you're both on the same side. Maybe you go about reaching your goals differently, and maybe your priorities are not exactly the same, but you aren't enemies, and you aren't plotting to do the other one in. When disagreements flare, try to put yourself in the other person's place, and remember; principles are rarely more important than people. If you seem to have reached an impasse, you may wish to consult with a trusted friend, counselor, or member of the clergy. Perhaps they will be able to help you get a different perspective.

If you level with family members, friends, and your boss about your *feelings,* instead of lecturing them or hoping they'll read your mind, they will be more likely to understand you and respect your decisions.

Remember that a series of small earth tremors relieves tension and pressure within the fault and often prevents a major earthquake. Likewise, if you handle each situation as it arises, you can relieve stress and tension in your relationships and perhaps prevent a major upheaval.

Techniques for Handling Your Thoughts

Many people who survive serious accidents, undergo major surgery, or narrowly escape death relive the events as though they had a videotape in their brain. Reviewing the details of tragic events is a normal mechanism for dealing with stress and grief. We use this process to desensitize ourselves and to come to terms with what happened. However, when our thoughts take over our lives, as they did Debbie W's., when they prevent us from moving ahead, we must yell "Stop!" out loud and shift to pleasant thoughts.

"When the RESOLVE group told me to stop ruminating over my lost baby by yelling 'Stop,' I thought people would think I was crazy," Debbie W. said. "But it worked. I finally convinced myself to live for the future instead of burying myself in the tragedy of my past. Now, instead of planning my baby's funeral, I'm decorating the nursery."

Prepare for Stressful Situations

You need to prepare yourself for stressful situations, even rehearse and practice for them. First, say to yourself:

- I am important.
- My opinions count.
- I have the right to say what I feel.

When the conflict begins, convince yourself to take the action you know is needed. Believe that what *you* want is important.

"I used to dread going to Sunday dinner at Mom's. My brother and his children always came and there was never a Sunday that someone didn't say, 'When are you going to give us a grandchild?' It had gotten to the point that my wife and I didn't want to see them again. But the RESOLVE group convinced me that my folks just didn't know they were hurting me and that I needed to level with them.

"I practiced what I wanted to say to them every day for a week, over and over, until I could say those words in my sleep: 'Mom, Dad, no one wants to give you a grandchild any more than Jan and I do. But right now we can't. We're doing everything we can to solve our problem. I know you don't mean to hurt us, but asking us when we're going to give you a grandchild only makes us feel like failures. We'd both appreciate your not saying any more about it.'

"You can't imagine how hard it was to tell my mom and dad that. But you know, they were really sorry. They had no idea they were hurting us. My dad apologized and Mom gave Jan a big hug. Now we look forward to spending Sunday with the folks."

How to Control Your Anger

Anger is a natural, healthy, nonevil emotion. Go ahead and get angry! Get it off your chest! But next time, why don't you lay some plans that will avoid an angry confrontation.

If you become angry, it's probably because you've given someone else the power to control you and your emotions. Remember, *you* are responsible for your feelings; others don't *make* you angry. How many times have you become angry when someone said:

"One of these days you'll pop up pregnant."

As someone puts her newborn in your arms: "You're going to have one of these someday."

"Isn't it about time for you to have children?"

"You'll just have to accept things."

"I don't understand why you do that to your body, just to have a baby. It isn't worth it."

Get to know yourself. Know what triggers your anger, what pushes your anger button. And don't set yourself up to get angry. Instead, plan some alternatives for these situations. If you know, for example, that holding a newborn baby drives you up the wall, be ready to say, "Oh, I'd better not hold her. I think I'm coming down with a cold." Or if you become uncomfortable at a dinner party, when someone you barely know asks you how many children you have, brush it off by saying, "We aren't quite ready to start our family yet."

You must remember that most people don't intend to cause you discomfort. And often they really aren't extremely interested in your answer; they're just making small talk. It's usually only because you are *listening defensively* that what they say gets to you. Getting angry is *your* problem, not theirs.

If someone repeatedly bothers you, a relative, for example, then you need to assert yourself and say, "Mother, you know it's unlikely that we're going to 'pop up pregnant' someday. You aren't cheering me up, you're making me feel worse. I'd appreciate your not saying things like that." Or, "We aren't ready to 'accept things.' As long as our doctor has hope, we aren't giving up. When you say things like that, I feel angry. I'd appreciate changing the subject."

Remember:

- Stick to specifics and to the present situation.
- Avoid generalizing and reviewing the entire history of your relationship.
- Deal with issues as they arise, when you feel your anger building.
- Work toward a resolution, not a victory.

Be honest with people, share your feelings with them, and don't put them on the defensive by making accusations. If they really care about you, they will do their best to help.

Learn to Fight Fair

It's okay to fight if you fight fair. Fair fights release tension and often lead to the resolution of problems. Unfair fights, though, create more tension and do not solve anything. To fight fair, you need to follow these rules:

- Do not tell your mate what he or she is thinking: "You don't really want this baby!" Instead, say how *you* are feeling: "Sometimes I'm not sure that you want this baby."
- Do not reach into the past for insults and injustices: "If you'd taken a semen analysis in the beginning, we'd be a year ahead of where we are now!" Instead, stick to the present: "Let's make an appointment to see the urologist."
- Do not resort to name-calling: "Your mother is a bitch!" Instead, look for solutions: "I believe it would be best for me to avoid long visits with your mother."

- Avoid a win/lose position: "I'm not changing my mind." Instead, seek understanding: "I feel very strongly about my position. I don't believe I can change my mind."

When Is It Time to Quit?

I wish I could give you a magic answer to this question: call a halt after two years, after in vitro, after adoption. But it's not that simple. There is no concrete answer that works for everyone.

Some people decide to take a breather from the rigors of fertility treatment: to stop taking their temperature, to stop taking medication, to stop worrying about whether they'll get pregnant this month. In fact, many even use birth control to prevent a pregnancy. After they've had some time to relax and to enjoy life, or after hearing of a new breakthrough in fertility treatment, they may once again renew their treatment efforts.

Other people want to make a final decision: they have a hysterectomy; they stop treatment and apply for adoption; they have their tubes tied. They want to get off the roller coaster forever and get on with their lives.

The best time to quit is when *you* decide to—not when you run out of money, not when others say it's all right, not when you've tried every possible treatment, not when you've hit bottom, but when *you* decide you want to quit.

As a couple, you must decide what "happy ending" will meet your needs. Will you be satisfied to remain childless? Will an adopted child meet your parenting needs? Will AID meet your needs? Will a surrogate mother meet your needs? Is an embryo transfer the answer? How much money are you comfortable spending? How much time will you devote to solving your fertility problem? Only when you've answered these questions *to your satisfaction* will you be able to move on with your life.

Two Special People

"What do you do when your spirits get low?" Shelley T. asked.

"Well, a good cry helps a lot!" Kathy S. smiled. "I've even been known to slam every door in the house!"

The group laughed.

"I appreciate the little things Bryan does to cheer me up," Debbie W. added. "After my second miscarriage he brought me breakfast in bed for a week. And every once in a while, for no special reason, he'll bring me a red rose."

"When we really get down, we splurge on something," Michael T. said. "It seems like we give up everything to pay for our fertility treatment. So even though we're careful to watch our budget, once in a while we do something special—go out to eat, go skiing, buy a new camera."

"Taking my temperature every morning used to get me down," Kathy said. "I hated to tell Steven, 'Today's the day.' It really helped when Steven started recording my temperature for me. Sharing the responsibility and making him aware of my fertile days took a lot of pressure off both of us."

"Let's face it, the stress we're under really strains our sexual desires and performance," Shelley said. "We really have trouble before a postcoital test."

"Ever since I realized I had a fertility problem, I haven't been able to enjoy sex—even during my so-called infertile days," Margaret B. said. "I've always been haunted by a lingering hope: maybe this time will be the time that works."

"Me, too," Kathy said. "But Steven always refuses to let our infertility get us down. I don't know what I would do without his positive attitude. Just when I'm at my lowest, he'll say, 'We're not going to let this thing stop our life.' "

Shelley said: "A couple I know sometimes uses birth control so they can enjoy sex. Because they know they *can't* get pregnant, neither of them feels that they must perform, and when her period starts, they don't feel they failed that month."

"It seems to me that infertility disturbs women more than it does men," Kathy said.

"At least we seem to show it more," Margaret said.

"I don't know about that," Shelley countered. "One time I thought Michael was going off the deep end. I didn't know what to do, so I called a RESOLVE member for help. She suggested that Michael talk to a RESOLVE husband having a similar fertility problem."

"Talking to Jerry was the best thing I ever did," Michael said.

"You know, that's really the key," Kathy said. "Having someone who will listen to you.

"Keeping our marriage together and learning again how to enjoy our sexuality hasn't been easy," Kathy added. "We've had to work hard at it, over many months." She reached for Steven's hand. "But it's been worth it." She smiled. "I don't mean to sound conceited, but I believe we have a stronger marriage than most of our friends, who have not gone through what we've had to."

You Have the Power to Change

Like these couples, you have the power to change your life. Change is hard work; it usually comes in small steps; not all at once. Always keep in mind that you can change only yourself and those things under your control, not others.

When you approach life assertively, fight fair, express your needs, accept responsibility for your feelings, and act openly and honestly—with yourself and with others—you will see the world through a new light. Armed with this knowledge and understanding about fertility treatment, you will be in control of your life and your future.

Keep your spirits up and know that you can do it. You are working with an infinitely valuable resource—*yourself*.

VI. Into the Future

21. High-Tech Babies: Now and in the Future

It's curious how my perspective has changed over the last ten or fifteen years. In medical school we were taught that it was theoretically possible to perform embryo transplants and genetic engineering. "But," I thought, "not in my lifetime." All of that has changed, since the birth of the first "test-tube baby" in 1978. With the monumental strides being made in genetics and our understanding of reproductive processes, I find myself wanting to offer these new discoveries to help my patients get their miracle babies.

I want, for example, to tell a twenty-nine-year-old patient who's having a hysterectomy that it's going to be okay. She can use her eggs, her husband's sperm, and a surrogate womb to have their own genetic baby. Or tell a forty-two-year-old woman who's been trying to get pregnant for nineteen years that she might be able to nurture a donor embryo. In some ways I feel that I am able to offer them new hope, but more often I feel frustrated by "the system" which deprives infertile couples of these opportunities.

In reflective moments I sometimes become concerned that we are tampering with people's lives in ways that violate basic human moralities. It's all happening so quickly, and yet there are so many barriers to hurdle—technical, sociological, ethical, and legal.

In this chapter I'd like to tell you about high-tech fertility treatment alternatives that are already available, such as artificial insemination and in vitro fertilization, and about the new technologies such as donor eggs, embryo transfer, and donor wombs *that we know work* but that we cannot freely recommend. Many of these options are not readily available because our scientific and medical advances have outstripped the ability of our society, religious beliefs, and laws to cope with their complexities. These issues, which I'll discuss, must be satisfactorily resolved before physicians can, in good conscience, offer technology's gifts.

Artificial Insemination

For years infertile couples have successfully taken advantage of artificial insemination (AI). The technique involves using a syringe to "artificially" squirt semen near the cervix or preferably directly inside the uterus (intrauterine artificial insemination, or IAIH). The nature of the fertility problem dictates whether the husband's sperm (artificial insemination homologous, or AIH) or a donor's sperm (artificial insemination donor, or AID) will be used.

Who Should Use Artificial Insemination?

The most obvious fertility problem requiring AI is poor semen quality. Often we can improve fertility by concentrating and/or washing a masturbated specimen and depositing the sperm next to the cervix. We can also inject them directly into the womb to bypass the cervical mucus. Intrauterine insemination with the husband's sperm (IAIH) will frequently solve a hostile sperm-mucus interaction or mucus quality problem.

Even if the man has as few as 5 to 10 million sperm per milliliter, there's still up to a 30 percent chance that IAIH will work. IAIH appears to be less effective in patients with low motility. Yet frequently a couple who has tried unsuccessfully for years will achieve a pregnancy using these rather simple techniques. The following summarizes the primary uses for IAIH:

Fertility Problems Resolved with IAIH

Small ejaculate volume	Large ejaculate volume
Low motility (less than 50%)	Poor sperm-mucus interaction
Coital disorder	Low sperm count
Unknown origin of infertility	Retrograde ejaculation

If AIH or IAIH fails, if the husband has no sperm, if the husband has a genetically transmitted disease, or if there is an Rh blood factor problem, donor sperm offers the couple an opportunity to have a child who is genetically related to the mother. Many couples prefer this alternative to adoption, since they can control the prenatal environment and the timing of the baby's arrival, avoid lengthy adoption procedures, and share the experience of pregnancy and birth.

In cases where the man is oligospermic, physicians may mix the husband's sperm with the donor's (AIM) so the couple doesn't really know whose sperm fertilized the egg. This procedure can degrade the donor semen, however, and jeopardize the results. Perhaps a better technique is for the couple to have intercourse the night following insemination—the aura of mystery will still exist.

With only 4 percent of teenage pregnancies being given up for adopton, AID offers hope to people who have waited unsuccessfully for adoption; and unlike adoption, AID involves very little red tape. Over twenty thousand U.S. couples use AID each year, and 57 percent of them succeed within three to six cycles. Here are some reasons why couples choose AID:

Fertility Problems Resolved with AID

Fertility Problem	% Solved with AID
Oligospermia (less than 20 million)	29–45
Azospermia (no sperm)	30–66
Vasectomy	8–30
Genetic problems with the man	1–4
Sexual disturbances	2
Systemic disease	1
Sperm autoimmunization/Rh isoimmunization	?

Technique for AI

Some doctors will encourage you to have your husband present to participate in the "special event." In the past we've primarily relied on the basal body temperature (BBT) chart to time AI to coincide with ovulation. Now, newer tests pinpoint ovulation more accurately. The First Response Ovulation Predictor Test from Tambrands Inc. is one of several inexpensive home tests that will predict your LH spike and ovulation. OvuSTICKS and Ovutime, which are somewhat more expensive than the Tambrands product, have proved to be quite reliable, too.

The CUE Fertility Monitor from Zetek* may also prove to be beneficial for predicting ovulation. I used the CUE monitor with Michael and Shelley T. to time AIH.

I reached into my desk drawer and pulled out a device the size of a hand calculator, with wires and probes hanging from it. "This is a CUE Fertility Monitor," I said, handing it to Shelley T. "I'm testing this for the manufacturer.

"For AIH to work, we have to know when you're going to ovulate. This device allows you to predict ovulation up to a week in advance.

"These small electrodes can sense minute changes in your body chemistry. Starting a week before you expect to ovulate, each morning you put the electrode in your mouth and record the digital display reading on this chart." I handed her the record sheet. "When the readings peak, we know that

*The CUE Fertility Monitor may be purchased directly from Zetek (Zetek, Inc., 794 Ventura Street, Aurora, CO 80011), or you may wish to lease it from your physician.

ovulation will occur in six days. To get a more precise measure, you then begin measuring the chemical changes in your vagina.

"Since you just finished your menstrual period, I'd like you to begin with the oral readings. We'll begin trying AIH next month. This monitor will be especially useful for predicting your fertile days."

If you do not ovulate the morning after you are inseminated, the procedure should be repeated one to two days later. The doctor will deposit the husband's or donor's semen near the cervix and have you stay prone for approximately thirty minutes. Some physicians will install a cervical cap to seal the sperm inside for four to six hours. (If you have intrauterine insemination, you do not need to remain prone; the sperm will not leak out of your uterus.)

Many physicians feel that even when the fertility problem appears to be solely the man's, the woman should have a tubal X ray before proceeding with AI treatment. If the woman does not appear to have a tubal problem and has no history of reproductive organ infection, I usually give her the option of delaying this procedure for three to four insemination tries. Not only is a hysterosalpingogram expensive and painful but it also carries the risk of introducing infection into the womb.

Sperm Banking

There are about twenty registered sperm banks in the United States. Half are associated with universities and medical schools. This should be comforting to potential AID users, since their most common concerns are that the donors be intelligent and healthy—traits one hopes to find in college and medical school populations. Donors must have a normal semen analysis, normal physical characteristics, and a negative history of genetic disease for three generations. Since sperm banks have large numbers of donors, almost any coloring, body type, blood type, and race can be matched. A *minimal* workup of the donor should include tests for hepatitis, VDRL, Tay-Sachs, ABO-Rh factors, white blood cells (infection), AIDS virus antibodies, chlamydia, gonorrhea, and mycoplasma. Homosexuals are not allowed to participate because of the risk of transmitting AIDS (acquired immune deficiency syndrome). A number of programs also eliminate known marijuana and drug users, since their sperm may lack motility. Not all banks screen black donors for sickle-cell anemia, though they should. Collected samples are frozen and stored for no more than three years.

Although with fresh semen collected in a doctor's office you may get pregnant in fewer cycles, many people prefer the safety of buying frozen specimens which have undergone better screening procedures. Moreover, the larger numbers of donors associated with sperm banks reduce the possibility of half brothers and half sisters marrying one day without knowing it. Sperm can be frozen and safely transported across the country, so AID can be available to you no matter where you live.

Potential Problems with AID

AID is not without its problems. Many people complain that the cattle industry does a far better job of screening donor bull sperm than sperm banks and physicians do. Although the cases are rare, AID has been linked to venereal disease being transmitted to the recipient, to babies born with genetically transmitted diseases, and to miscarriages from genetic abnormalities. And now with the AIDS virus threat, many physicians and their patients will be even more apprehensive about donor screening procedures. Tracing the problem to a specific donor may be impossible, since many physicians mix sperm from different donors (to protect anonymity) or keep inadequate records. I do not recommend mixing sperm because I feel it is very important for the child to have access to his or her genetic history.

Because of their lowered fertility potential, women with endometriosis, a history of pelvic disease, and ovulatory problems do not respond as well to AI as others. In addition, women over thirty years old have a 30 percent lower pregnancy rate than younger women.

Only half of the states recognize the legitimacy of an AID baby. Many religions forbid masturbation (necessary for AIH) and also condemn the use of donor sperm—some even claim it to be adultery. Although your state law may require you to obtain court consent for AID, there are no laws that forbid AID—even to an unmarried woman. You may wish to check with an attorney to see how you can protect your child's inheritance rights and your paternity rights upon death or divorce.

Is AID Right for You?

When husbands learn that they are infertile, about 80 percent of them have guilt feelings. They often feel unworthy and incapable in many other areas of their lives. For up to three months following the diagnosis nearly two-thirds lose their sex drive or become impotent. Wives frequently become angry with their husbands, though not directly because of their fertility problem. Within two to three months nearly half of these couples experience severe marital difficulties. But they seldom link the problem to the husband's diagnosis.

Even if you desperately want a child, no one should rush into AID. In fact, some countries have mandatory waiting periods of from three to six months between the diagnosis of a man's infertility and implementation of the AID procedure. During this time the couple can discuss their concerns, explore the pros and cons, and adjust to the idea that he will never genetically father a child. Working through these problems keeps the wife from being caught between *his failure* to impregnate her and *her success* at pregnancy with another man's sperm.

When asked, about one-third of men who choose to use AID feel pressured by their wives to do so, whereas only 6 percent of wives felt pressured by their husbands. Some wives will even threaten divorce if the husband will not allow them to have an AID baby. Apparently, though, AID couples develop stronger marriages than most people, because their divorce rate is only 1 percent, compared with an overall divorce rate of 49.6 percent.

Having made the decision to use AID, between 25 and 40 percent of the couples will drop out of the program due to the stress of taking temperatures, regulating cycles, and so forth. Some, however, will return to try again later.

If you use AID, you will have to decide whether friends, grandparents, and other relatives should know where the baby came from. Since doctors can match the traits of the donor to those of the husband (coloring, stature, etc.) and the same donor may be used for several children, many people would never suspect that the husband did not father the children. In the past about 85 percent of AID users never told anyone. In light of recent advancements in organ transplants and genetic counseling, which will reveal a person's genetic heritage, the trend toward secrecy may reverse—the child may need to know his or her true genetic heritage. It may be unfair, for example, for a son to worry about developing heart disease because his father died of it, when, in fact, the son was conceived with AID and is not genetically related to him.

When You Consent to AID

If you use AID, the wife and many times the husband must sign an informed consent form. Your doctor should cover the following information when discussing the procedure with you:

AID Informed Consent

Risks and consequences of the AID procedures the doctor uses
Information on the donor:
    How donors are selected
    Medical/genetic history of the donor
    Tests given to donors
    Tests run on the donor's semen
    Records kept on donor
    Information disclosure on donor (physician's or clinic's policy and state
      law)
Other semen tests which you could request to minimize risks
Risks that cannot be screened for
Risks of pregnancy
State law may require that a married woman have husband's consent.

Decisions for the Future

Physicians have faced some rather difficult decisions about artificial insemination: What if a single woman or a lesbian wants AID? At first many physicians resisted this practice; however, since all states allow unmarried people to adopt and no law forbids AID to single women, the woman has the upper hand. Currently, one in ten practitioners will perform AID for her, without setting qualifications such as employment, ability to support the child, and so forth.

What if a couple wants to freeze the husband's sperm before he goes into the armed forces? Has dangerous surgery? Undergoes radiation treatments? Should he die, who "owns" his sperm? Can the widow use the deceased husband's sperm to bear him a legitimate heir? Doctors and lawyers are grappling with these problems. Many must simply follow their own conscience or make a best guess at what a court might do, should it come to that.

Before most existing state laws will recognize the legitimacy of the child, a doctor must prescribe AID. Some people speculate, however, that using donor sperm will become so acceptable and commonplace that you'll be able to purchase semen directly in the form of a home kit. Who knows what they'll come up with? Maybe it will be freeze-dried.

In Vitro Fertilization

In vitro fertilization became a reality with the birth of Louise Brown, the first "test-tube baby," on July 24, 1978, after years of research and painstaking work by Drs. Robert Edwards and Patrick Steptoe in Oldham, England. The techniques were brought to the United States by Howard Jones, who, with his wife, Georgeanna, operates an in vitro clinic at East Virginia Medical School. Today there are over one hundred in vitro clinics in the United States and several hundred elsewhere in the world.

Who Should Use In Vitro Fertilization?

In vitro fertilization was originally developed to bypass nonfunctional or absent fallopian tubes, but now we realize that the procedure also offers opportunities to couples with prolonged, unexplained fertility problems and to men with low sperm counts (under 20 million). The procedure involves retrieving matured eggs from the ovaries, fertilizing them in a petri dish with a masturbated sperm specimen (husband's or donor's), and transferring the dividing embryo into the uterus for implantation.

In a collaborate report from in vitro fertilization and embryo replacement clinics from around the world, as of January 1984, sixty-five teams had retrieved eggs from a total of 7,993 cycles leading to the birth of 600 infants—

an overall live birthrate of 10 percent per month compared with a normal fertility rate of 20 percent per month. There were 457 single births, 57 twins (10.9 percent), 7 triplets (1.3 percent), and 2 quadruplets. During this same time period there were 324 clinical abortions and 19 ectopic pregnancies. Half of the babies were delivered by cesarean section. As might be expected, the best results came from women under thirty years old—13.6 percent. Women over forty, who are normally less fertile than younger women, averaged 7.2 percent. In addition, the pregnancy rates increased considerably with the transfer of multiple embryos: one embryo resulted in a 9.7 percent success, two embryos 14.6 percent, three embryos 19.3 percent, and four or more embryos 24.1 percent. And to everyone's great relief, none of the babies born had chromosomal abnormalities!

Although the findings are not conclusive, there seems to be a reduced success rate with severe endometriosis, unexplained infertility, abnormal semen analysis, and sperm antibody problems with either the man or the woman.

Many in vitro clinics will eliminate "less desirable" applicants: you can be denied these services because of a history of genetically transferred disease in your family, because of your age (over thirty-five, for example), because of your weight, because of uterine abnormalities, or because you have abnormal menstrual cycles. Due to differing state laws, many in vitro clinics will not consider using donor sperm at this time. The issue of single women or lesbians requesting in vitro fertilization with donor sperm is just now being considered.

Techniques for In Vitro Fertilization

The Workup

Most clinics will do a complete fertility workup before accepting you for the in vitro program. Some, however, will accept fertility records from your own physician. Only after they are certain that conventional fertility treatment options have been exhausted and that you have a reasonable expectation for success will they enroll you in the in vitro program.

The woman's workup will include an interview, screening laparoscopy (if there are tubal factors), a pelvic examination, an ultrasound examination of the uterus, and routine laboratory tests. The husband will receive a standard semen analysis as well as tests for immunologic factors, bacteria culture, and egg penetration.

Stimulating Egg Growth

Since success rates increase with multiple embryo transfers, most clinics will stimulate the woman's ovaries to produce a number of mature follicles. Between cycle days 2 and 5 you will begin taking oral Serophene or Pergonal injections for five consecutive days to stimulate follicular development. (See chapter 14 for more details on ovulation induction.) Daily ultrasound and blood tests (to test LH and estrogen levels) will tell the doctor when your follicles are mature enough for harvesting. Around day 11 or 12 you will receive an hCG injection to prepare the eggs for release. Prior to your ovulating, however, the doctor will retrieve the eggs from the follicles. Today two methods are being used for egg retrieval: laparoscopy and ultrasound.

Laparoscopic Egg Retrieval

Laparoscopy is done with the woman under general anesthesia. The doctor inserts the laparoscope (small telescope) through a small incision in your belly button. A suction needle is inserted through a tiny hole just above your pubic bone. The doctor inflates your abdomen with carbon dioxide to uncover the ovaries for the retrieval operation. One by one the doctor punctures the bulging follicles and gently suctions out their precious cargo. Specially trained technicians transfer each egg to its own specially prepared petri dish. Bathed in nutritious broth and warmed in an incubator, the eggs continue to mature while the mother recovers from the egg retrieval procedure. Mature eggs are allowed to incubate for six to eight hours; immature eggs for twenty-six hours.

Ultrasound Egg Retrieval

Some clinics are using a new ultrasound retrieval procedure developed in England and Germany. Instead of using the laparoscope, the doctor uses ultrasound to locate the bulging follicles. Since the doctor retrieves the eggs with a long needle inserted through the vagina, abdominal wall, or bladder, the procedure is relatively painless and does not require general anesthesia.

Ultrasonic retrieval can be performed in a doctor's office at far less cost than laparoscopic egg retrieval. The egg retrieval, fertilization, and pregnancy rates compare favorably with laparoscopic results.

Collecting the Semen

Two hours before the insemination the husband, who has been asked to abstain for three to five days prior to the procedure, collects a fresh semen sample. The sperm are washed and treated so they can penetrate the egg. If the man's count is under 20 million, the sperm will be centrifuged and concentrated. Although clinic practices vary, it seems that only 50,000 to 200,000 sperm are needed to fertilize each egg, as compared with over 20 million in nature. (Some clinics claim they need only a hundred or so sperm to fertilize the egg.)

In Vitro Fertilization

The sperm are placed in the dish (in vitro or in glass) for fertilization. The mixture then returns to the incubator until the embryo divides into four to eight cells. The best transfer results seem to occur forty to forty-four hours after insemination. At this point in the procedure most clinics are 75 to 95 percent successful.

Preparing the Uterus for Implantation

While the embryos incubate, the woman receives a progesterone injection to prepare her uterus for implantation. To avoid infection, the woman also receives tetracycline twenty-four hours before and after the transfer.

Embryo Transfer

The embryo transfer process is exciting for everyone present—husband, wife, doctor, and assistants. The doctor slips a catheter into the woman's cervix and injects the embryos into her uterus. She is advised to remain quiet for two to three days to allow time for the embryos to acclimate to their new environment, where at least one, it is hoped, will be implanted.

Gamete Intrafallopian Transfer (GIFT)

An exciting new transfer technique may offer better results for those women with functional tubes and men with poor semen. After retrieving the eggs by laparoscopy, they are placed in a long tube together with the sperm. Then the physician transfers the mixture through the fallopian tube end (fimbria) for in vivo (in the living body) fertilization and implantation.

Initial results show GIFT to be as effective as in vitro techniques, and it is much less expensive. GIFT may also prove valuable in resolving unexplained infertility.

Pregnancy

A positive pregnancy test brings joy to everyone; however, the couple isn't out of the woods yet. Over half of these "chemical pregnancies" terminate prematurely. To support the uterine lining, many doctors prescribe progesterone suppositories until the pregnancy is confirmed, and progesterone injections until the second trimester. However, even in the best of circumstances, 33 percent of the embryos will spontaneously abort within the first twelve weeks, and 10 to 15 percent will abort later. This 50 percent abortion rate, twice as high as the normal rate, reduces the chances for having a term baby to 10 percent.

Delivery

Some in vitro programs automatically deliver all babies by cesarean section, but I believe that unless the pregnancy and delivery warrant this surgical procedure, a vaginal delivery should be attempted.

Potential Problems

A number of technical problems may arise during the in vitro procedure: the laparoscopy may cause an infection in the woman so the transfer procedure must be canceled; the man may not be able to masturbate on command (sometimes the woman, recovering from general anesthesia, must help him with this task); or the sperm may not fertilize the eggs. These problems, however, are infrequent.

Some doctors feel that the high abortion rate may be due in part to the effects of the ovulation induction hormones, anesthesia, and retrieval procedures. Researchers speculate that freezing the embryos and transferring them later, during a "normal" cycle, will improve the success rates. They also point out that, should the first transfer not implant, extra embryos (over the three or four transplanted in the first procedure) could be saved for subsequent cycles. The frozen embryos could also be saved for initiating subsequent pregnancies. Embryo freezing would reduce the number of laparoscopies and egg retrieval procedures the woman must go through. Although strict embryo experimentation laws in some states often forbid embryo freezing, we're beginning to see some changes that will make these procedures available in the near future.

When You Consent to In Vitro

You will be asked to sign an informed consent form in order to receive in vitro services. The physician should explain the following information:

In Vitro Informed Consent

How the in vitro procedure will be performed
Any dangers with laparoscopy, anesthesia, and transfer procedures
Increased risks for birth defects
Measures taken to detect birth defects
Usual risks of pregnancy
Procedures used to dispose of fertilized ova not implanted
If donor sperm is used, AID informed consent (see page 230)

Decisions for the Future

Many people feel it's unfair to put a "healthy" woman through the rigors of in vitro fertilization—the risks to her health, the emotional stress, and so forth—because her husband has a poor sperm count. Many clinics will also tie off her normal fallopian tubes as a precaution against ectopic pregnancy.

Critics point out that with AID the woman could have a baby without an operation and at far less risk and cost, even though the baby would not be her husband's genetic heir. Others feel that this choice should be left to the couple.

Many religious groups and others oppose in vitro fertilization because they feel it interferes with "nature" or "God's Plan." They feel that if society doesn't put some limit on manipulating human life, things will get out of control—and there may be some merit to their concerns. For example, while the fertilized eggs are incubating in the laboratory, one day we might be able to examine the chromosomes and eliminate not only genetic abnormalities (Down's syndrome, sickle-cell anemia, Tay-Sachs disease, etc.) but also girl babies or boy babies.

Should a couple be able to "abort" the girl embryos because they want a son? Should the couple be able to "abort" the boy embryos if a sex-linked genetic disease runs in the family? Or, when our genetic engineering techniques become sophisticated enough, should the couple be able to select embryos based on other traits, such as eye and hair color? Even more dramatically, should they be able to alter the embryo's natural gene structure—by borrowing genes from donor chromosomes, for example?

And what of the fate of the unused fertilized embryo? Currently most in vitro programs fertilize only the three or four healthiest-looking eggs and transfer only the *dividing* embryos to the mother. Is it right to destroy the others? In Australia the mother can choose to freeze her extra embryos and/ or donate them to another woman. Now, that conjures up a whole bag of questions about "adopted embryos." We'll talk more about them later. But what happens if the mother or father dies, leaving frozen embryos in a tissue bank? Does someone inherit the embryos? Do the embryos have a right to life? To the parents' inheritance? Recently a judge in Australia said no to just such a case, and the embryos were destroyed.

Researchers say they could improve in vitro procedures and reduce miscarriages if they could observe the embryo developing for longer periods of time. However, current laws prevent this much-needed human embryo research. Even with the donor's consent, researchers must stop human embryo experiments after the fourteenth day of gestation. It's at this time that the embryo's nervous system begins to form (differentiate).

In contrast, successful breeding practices developed through embryo research in the cattle industry promise some exciting possibilities. We know, for example, that once the fertilized egg divides, we can separate the two cells and create identical twins. This is done routinely to maximize the fertility potential of prize cows. Each twin is then transferred to a surrogate mother, thus doubling the prize cow's fertility potential. What if a couple, using this technique, chose to transfer one twin and freeze the second twin for a future pregnancy? If the first twin turned out all right, the second twin could be born several years later.

Should society allow scientists to experiment with human life? Some feel that left unchecked, scientists may attempt to breed cross species (half animal and half man—chimera). Or they may create a human clone by removing the fertilized egg's genetic material and substituting chromosomes from two sperm. The baby might have a father and no mother. Or possibly a mother and no father. Others feel that eugenics programs will evolve and selectively eliminate many characteristics from the human race. Unfortunately, selective breeding for a "superior race" is not a new or untried idea.

Others fear that human reproduction may become a mechanized, impersonalized laboratory procedure. As a form of birth control, people might be sterilized routinely after having frozen several embryos. Then when they are ready for a family, they will report to the cryogenic tissue bank to receive their frozen embryo. Others see these options as insurance against tragedy: frozen embryos stored safely in a tissue bank would provide a backup should the man or woman become sterile from exposure to toxic substances, from an injury, or from illness or surgery.

Regardless of what you think about the advantages or threats posed by in vitro fertilization and human embryo research, it has become a new fact of life. As doctors, as infertile couples, and as a society, we're all going to have to deal with this reality.

Many infertile couples view in vitro fertilization as their last resort. Today perhaps it does stand as high tech's final answer. Yet even more spectacular possibilities lie in the not too distant future.

Embryo (Egg) Transfers

Embryo transfers began in 1972 in the cattle industry as a way of maximizing the fertility of prize cattle. By superovulating the best cows in the herd and transferring multiple embryos to cows of lesser breeding, one prize cow could pass her genes to many calves each year. One of the main problems that had to be overcome was synchronizing all of the surrogates to the menstrual cycle of the donor. But successful embryo freezing techniques resolved that difficulty. Ranchers could also twin embryos to double the harvest and discard the unwanted male embryos. Some have gone so far as to suggest that other species could be used as surrogate mothers; for example, a prize race horse could gestate in a donkey uterus.

Embryo transfer, or egg transfer as it's frequently called, is the female counterpart of donor artificial insemination (AID). Instead of the woman receiving donor sperm, however, she receives either a donor egg or, more likely, an embryo created with her husband's sperm and a donor egg.

Up to this point the only hope for restoring fertility to these couples was an ovary transplant. To date, however, organ transplants have restored fertility in only a few isolated cases. With the advances in in vitro procedures, it's doubtful that the risks of major surgery and organ rejection (except with identical twins) justify these extraordinary measures.

We are much more likely to solve these female fertility problems with donor eggs (oocytes) and embryos. Eggs might be retrieved from women anticipating pelvic surgery, for example, or from volunteer egg donors. TDO (transfer of donor oocytes) also resolves several legal complications. The law views the woman carrying the pregnancy (gestation mother) as the legal mother; and egg manipulation does not fall under the stringent rules associated with fetal (embryo) research. The doctor would need to obtain consent only from the donor and recipient.

Who Should Use Embryo Transfers?

Women with nonfunctional or no ovaries and women with a family history of genetic disease can benefit from donor embryos, as may women failing in vitro procedures or having some forms of unexplained infertility and recurrent abortions. It's also possible that unresolved sperm antibody problems could be overcome by using the husband's sperm with a donor egg.

Embryo transfer offers a number of benefits: the husband will have an opportunity to be genetically related to the baby; the couple can share the pregnancy and birth; and uterine bonding will occur with the mother. As with AID, there are no lengthy adoption procedures or waiting periods. However, even though embryo transfer has been successfully used to initiate several pregnancies, few clinics will attempt the procedure because of potential legal complications and social pressures.

Technique for Embryo Transplants

Rather than harvest the donor eggs with laparoscopy or ultrasound monitoring retrieval procedures, a simpler method is used. The doctor can inseminate the donor with the husband's sperm and four to five days later attempt to wash the embryo from her womb and transfer the embryo through a catheter into the wife's womb. Until human embryo freezing is accepted, this procedure requires that both women's cycles be synchronized with medications. Neither woman, however, faces the risks of anesthesia or surgery, and pain is very minimal.

Limited experience with humans shows that transplants have succeeded in 16.7 percent of the cases, approaching the normal fertility rates of 20 percent per cycle. Since the success rate in animal breeding is quite good, many researchers expect that with experience the rate will approach one-third.

Potential Problems with Embryo Transplants

The uterine washing technique (lavage) and transfer process may cause an ectopic pregnancy or infection in either woman. In addition, the donor always risks the possibility that the embryo will resist lavage and implant in her uterus, and she'll end up with an unwanted pregnancy. In this situation she must either choose to carry the baby to term or have an elective abortion. Either of these options may compromise the father's rights and the donor's health. The infertile couple may grieve for their aborted baby or might want to adopt the baby if it is carried to term. In addition, the donor may risk contracting a venereal disease from the artificial insemination process.

Since the egg is fertilized in vivo (in the living body of the donor), artificial embryonation (AE) falls outside embryo experimentation laws. Since the flushing technique comes under the abortion laws, there is no legal problem as long as the procedure is performed with the donor's consent. And since the law views the gestational mother as the legal mother, custody and adoption complications are averted.

Decisions for the Future

Certain couples object to embryo transfer because the uterine lavage is essentially an abortion. Some of their objections could be avoided by retrieving the donor's eggs and using the in vitro fertilization procedures described earlier in this chapter. It's unlikely, however, that many donors will submit to these surgical procedures.

Our society and legal system have not addressed the issues that embryo transfers raise. For example, will the definition of "illegitimate child" be broadened to include a child born to a woman who used her husband's sperm and another woman's egg? Will the man be guilty of adultery if his sperm fertilizes another woman's egg for his wife's pregnancy? Sounds like fertile fodder for lawyers and theologians. (Pardon the pun.)

Donor selection may be problematic. Should the donor be anonymous, or a friend or relative? Should the donor have physical characteristics and intelligence similar to the gestational mother? And how will the donor be screened for genetic abnormalities, infection, and so forth? It's likely that egg donors will be selected in much the same way as AID donors.

For embryo transfer to become a popular option, the donors will have to be paid for their services (as are AID donors). Since the embryo donor must go through artificial insemination and lavage procedures, and increase her risk for having an ectopic pregnancy, she'll undoubtedly want more compensation. One clinic reportedly paid donors $250 per cycle, and another paid $50 per egg retrieved and $200 for each fertilized egg retrieved. Will this payment be interpreted as baby selling?

Arrangements will also have to be made to handle accidental donor pregnancies and treatment for complications such as ectopic pregnancy and infection. In addition, the rights of the father must be clarified should the donor decide to carry an implanted pregnancy to term.

Some people feel that embryo freezing techniques may someday offer couples an opportunity for prenatal adoption: donor egg plus donor sperm.

Instead of arranging for embryo transfer, couples will be able to "purchase" an embryo much as they do sperm today—or will they? Will they still have to pass rigorous, lengthy qualifying "adoption" procedures to get an embryo? And who will qualify? Will you have to prove infertility? Will you have to be employed? Will you have to be heterosexual and married? Will you have to be under a certain age? If you buy frozen sperm and frozen egg separately (not a fertilized embryo), will these restrictions still apply? Many questions will have to be answered.

Embryo transfer is even more exciting than artificial insemination was only a few years ago. I wouldn't be surprised if donor embryos became readily available to infertile couples before 1990.

Surrogate Mothers

When Rose C. had her complete hysterectomy at age twenty-seven, she and Nick lost all hope of ever having their own child. After recovering from their grief, they decided to apply for adoption. They'd been on the waiting list for several years with three different agencies and were about to give up when a close friend offered an interesting possibility:

"Why don't you let me have your child for you?" Marcie said. "I don't have any trouble getting pregnant. In fact, I rather enjoy it."

Rose couldn't believe what she was hearing. "Are you serious?"

"I wouldn't suggest it if I weren't. Look, it's tearing me up seeing you moping around. When I was pregnant with Aaron, you didn't say anything, but I could tell that even though you were happy for me, you were miserable. All I did was remind you of your hysterectomy."

"But how could I ask you to have my child for me?" Rose's eyes filled with tears.

"Come on, we've been friends ever since I can remember. We'd do anything for each other. Why don't you let me do this for you and Nick. It's the greatest gift I could give you."

These couples did work out a wonderful solution to Nick and Rose C.'s fertility problem. They found a doctor who would inseminate Marcie with Nick's sperm. On the second try Marcie conceived and nine months later presented them with their new son, Christopher. Both couples attended the home birth; in fact, they made a videotape of the momentous occasion. Afterward Marcie and her husband relinquished their parental rights and, to make things legal, Nick and Rose C. adopted Christopher.

Unfortunately not all surrogate relationships end this happily. Using friends or relatives may be an emotional time bomb. Moreover, because surrogate contracts are not recognized by the courts, the prospective parents and the surrogate donor can encounter many legal difficulties.

Who Should Use a Surrogate Mother?

If a woman cannot carry a pregnancy, a surrogate mother may provide the couple with an opportunity to have a child. Because of additional costs and the rigors of in vitro procedures, Nick and Rose C. chose to use a surrogate. Christopher was genetically related to Nick. (With in vitro fertilization the possibility also arises that the child could be genetically related to both the mother and the father. For example, since Rose C. still had her ovaries, the doctor could have harvested her eggs, fertilized them in vitro with Nick's sperm, and transferred the embryo to Marcie's womb. Marcie would have nurtured and given birth to Nick and Rose C.'s baby.)

Women who have no uterus, have no ovaries, who don't respond to ovulation induction therapy, who carry a genetic disease, or who have health problems that preclude pregnancy could benefit from surrogate arrangements. Some people even suggest that women who cannot safely carry pregnancies due to occupational hazards could benefit from a surrogate.

The Surrogate Procedure

The technique is rather simple. The traditional method is to use the husband's sperm to artificially inseminate the surrogate mother. If the couple wants to use the wife's eggs, the doctor would synchronize the women's cycles, stimulate the wife to ovulate, retrieve her eggs, fertilize them in vitro with her husband's sperm, and transfer the embryo into the surrogate. (If they used frozen embryos, cycle synchronization could be avoided. At present, however, embryo transfer to a surrogate is not done in the United States.)

Surrogate relationships usually cost between $5,000 and $20,000, including medical and legal expenses. If the surrogate lives in a different state or town, some travel may be involved for the inseminations, for the birth, and for bringing the baby home.

Most surrogate contracts will specify that the surrogate agree to amniocentesis to check the child for genetic disease and to paternity testing to ensure that the couple is getting the child they paid for. In addition, the contract may insist that the surrogate agree to an abortion should the amniocentesis reveal a serious disorder.

The surrogate relationship, however, can be complex and psychologically exhausting.

Potential Problems

No one should rush into a surrogate relationship. The couple will experience a great deal of stress and worry throughout the pregnancy, so the marriage should have a firm foundation before any action is taken. They should make sure that the wife can accept a child born of another woman and will not feel inadequate because another woman can conceive with her husband's sperm while she cannot.

Our laws do not recognize surrogate relationships, surrogate contracts, or paternal claims to the baby. And should the wife's egg be used, she would have no claim, since there's no such thing as a "maternity suit" (not yet, anyway).

The first barrier facing the couple, however, is finding a surrogate mother. In Nick and Rose C.'s case the surrogate happened to be a lifelong friend. This turned into a very good relationship for them all. But it could just as easily have destroyed their friendship: What if Marcie drank too much alcohol and the parents became concerned about the fetus's welfare? What if Marcie didn't see her gynecologist regularly or take her maternity vitamins? What if Marcie wanted a home birth and Nick and Rose wanted their baby born in a hospital?

Many couples who do not know the surrogate or who live far away from the surrogate worry constantly about how she is taking care of the baby. They fear that the surrogate may back out of the contract and keep the baby for herself. Some couples are concerned about the possibility that the surrogate may have had sexual relations with her husband or boyfriend and the baby may not be a product of the insemination. Adoptive parents don't experience this anxiety because they don't know until they get a phone call that a baby is actually waiting for them.

The couple, an attorney, or an agency may select the surrogate. The couple may specify body type and may even be able to review pictures and biographical sketches of possible candidates. Some couples schedule an anonymous meeting with the surrogate. Most people feel that anonymity is important for protecting the family and child from future encounters with the surrogate. Anonymity also relieves the couple of feelings that they are obligated to keep in touch with the surrogate. However, many couples feel that establishing rapport with the surrogate may improve their chances that the surrogate will give the child up to them after its birth.

To help with the trauma associated with maternal separation, some arrangements will prevent the surrogate mother from seeing the baby after birth. Other contracts provide for the couple to attend the child's birth so all can share in the joy together.

The best surrogates, it seems, should have a moderate financial motive. On the one hand, if they are desperate for money, they may use the baby to blackmail the couple; on the other hand, if money is not a motive, they may decide to keep the child. The surrogate should have no history of genetic disease, alcoholism, heavy smoking, depression, or chronic physical disease. Many people feel that if the surrogate already has children she'll understand better what giving up a child will really mean. In addition, if the surrogate has a support system in place—for example, a husband or mother who condones the process—she'll be more likely to surrender the baby. No one knows for sure, however, if the surrogate will honor the contract and give the child to the couple—and the courts will probably stand behind the surrogate's decision, since at this time the woman who carries the pregnancy is seen as the legal mother.

Many feel that "renting" a surrogate womb is far less complex than "renting her womb and her genes, too." If the child belongs genetically to the infertile couple (husband's sperm plus wife's egg), the surrogate will be less likely to feel that her own baby is growing in her womb. So embryo transfers to surrogates may be preferable to artificially inseminating the surrogate.

Since the contracting couple must adopt the child, the adoption laws in the state where the surrogate resides play a big role. In states where all adoptions must go through a state agency adoption may be impossible. Many state laws stipulate that if the surrogate's husband consents to the insemination, he is the legal father. Other state laws presume that the surrogate's husband is the legal father no matter what and will not allow paternity blood tests as evidence to the contrary—even if the surrogate's husband has had a vasectomy! Other states require a mandatory waiting period before an adoption can take place.

States with stepparent adoption laws offer the least difficulty. In this situation the husband claims paternity from the outset. When the surrogate relinquishes her parental rights to the legitimate father, then his wife can adopt the stepchild (even though with embryo transfer the child is genetically hers). This arrangement not only does away with the waiting period and adoption suitability investigation but also clarifies another major issue: payments to the surrogate.

Baby selling is illegal. And paying a surrogate more than her medical expenses could be considered baby selling or paying her for relinquishing the baby for adoption. However, if the husband acknowledges paternity, he may be able to claim that the payments are to support the woman whom he impregnated . . . or that the payments are to have her relinquish parental rights, for putting the child up for adoption . . . well, it gets pretty complicated, as you can see.

The other questions that arise are: What happens if the contracting couple change their mind, divorce, or die during the pregnancy? What happens if the baby aborts? Who is responsible if the baby is born with a deformity or mental retardation? What happens if the surrogate does not keep her side of the bargain and jeopardizes the health of the fetus? And who gives permission for costly lifesaving emergency medical attention that the newborn might require? If you feel the emergency measures for newborn or surrogate were due to the surrogate's negligence, who pays?

The Roman Catholic Church views the surrogate relationship as adulterous and defines it as baby selling. The other major religions have no official position.

When You Consent to a Surrogate Relationship

Before a physician will assist with a surrogate mother relationship, all three parties—husband, wife, and surrogate—have to sign an informed consent. The physician should discuss the following issues:

Surrogate Mother Informed Consent

The AID informed consent information for surrogate (see page 230)
How surrogate is selected
Screening procedures used for surrogate: health, intelligence, emotional stability, genetics, physical characteristics, etc.
Further tests that can be done to identify other risks
Risks that cannot be screened for
Potential legal difficulties involved in entering a surrogate mother contract and with adoption procedures (state law)

Decisions for the Future

Some people are concerned about who should be permitted to hire a surrogate and for what reasons: Can a homosexual couple hire a surrogate to have their baby? Can a woman executive hire a surrogate so she won't have to interrupt her career? Can a single man hire a surrogate so he won't have to marry to have a child?

Society must decide if surrogate mothers offer a vital service to infertile couples, if surrogate mothering is a respectable occupation—a legitimate way to supplement the family income—or if surrogate mothers are selling their bodies much as prostitutes do. Others fear that fertilized embryos will be transferred to "breeders"—perhaps women imported from underdeveloped countries who need the financial support. If surrogate mothering is to work, then we must change our laws to protect the parties involved. We also need to protect the legitimacy and the rights of babies who would not have had an opportunity for life without this miraculous technological breakthrough.

Where Are We Headed?

Some people believe that once we begin tampering with human life, there will be no end to our lust for power and control over these most basic biological processes. Instead of seeing progress in embryology and genetic engineering as an opportunity to improve our quality of life, they see us destroying female fetuses in favor of males, manipulating human genetics to breed a superbaby, and degrading the precious, loving moments of creation, pregnancy, and birth into breeding farms.

These same people are concerned about the pressures that might be brought to bear on parents who are not infertile, but who could "improve" their offspring by using donor genes. Will a son or daughter be pressured by in-laws to use donor gametes so the grandbaby won't have a large nose or acne? Will a mother who sees herself as plain and homely want her daughter to have an opportunity to be beautiful? Will a man who always felt inadequate because he was small want his son to be six feet tall and have a muscular physique? Should people have to face these pressures and defend their decisions? Many people don't want their children and grandchildren to have to make these choices.

I guess I have more faith in the human race than most of these skeptics. We've proved time and time again that we can act responsibly—that we can control our knowledge and use it for the "good" of humankind. I do feel we should proceed cautiously, however, to prevent people from being conned into thinking that if they place themselves in the hands of fertility treatment specialists, all their problems will be solved. People must know the potential risks, they must have a realistic concept about their odds for success, and they must be counseled about the rigors of treatment regimens and the social pressures and legal entanglements they may encounter.

I hope that my discussion of this material has given you some insight into what's available and what's soon to come. With this knowledge you can decide whether or not to lobby for legislative changes, to support research projects, or to work toward changing public opinion. And you will be better prepared to discuss these issues with each other, your doctors, lawyers, family, friends, and clergy.

Epilogue

One of the advantages of being an obstetrician-gynecologist is that I can not only help my fertility patients achieve pregnancy but I can also deliver the fruit of our efforts.

Recently four RESOLVE couples invited me to a special kind of reunion— one to celebrate the resolution of their fertility problem.

As I walked into the restaurant, I wondered why, over the telephone, Kathy S. had been so mysterious about who would be joining us.

"Hi, Doctor."

I wove my way through the crowd to our table. As I looked around it, I recognized Bryan and Debbie W., Richard and Margaret B., Michael and Shelley T., Kathy and Steven S.—and four bright-eyed babies.

"Well, *they* wouldn't be here if it weren't for you," Kathy S. said.

"Besides," Margaret B. said, "we waited so long to get them, we wouldn't *think* of leaving them home."

Richard pulled a chair out from the head of the table. "You're our guest of honor," he said.

"Who is that?" I asked as I slipped into the chair. I was looking at a beautiful, plump, blue-eyed toddler.

"She's ours," Debbie said proudly. "She was only four pounds three ounces when you saw her last."

I remembered how concerned Debbie had been about losing another pregnancy. After I secured her weakened cervix, we both kept our fingers crossed, and as each month passed we became more and more excited about winning the battle. When she entered her eighth month without having gone into premature labor, we knew we were home free.

I smiled. "Looks just like her mother." Babbling noises to my right drew my attention to a little girl surrounded by lacy, yellow ruffles. "And who is this? Let me guess. It's got to be Jamie. She's got her father's eyes."

247

"Right," Steven said. "And her mother's spunk."

Steven was right about that. Kathy did have spunk. AIH hadn't been a picnic for Steven either. He had really been supportive. If they hadn't stuck with their fertility treatment plan as they did, Jamie would still be a dream.

"And look who we've got." Shelley plucked a tiny blue bundle from a carrier and pulled the blanket aside. "This is Tommy's first adventure out of the house. We just got him from the agency two days ago."

"Tell us what happened," Kathy demanded.

"I was just sitting there Monday afternoon and the phone rang. I thought it was my mother calling, but it was the agency. She said, 'We have a three-week-old baby boy who needs a home. Are you still interested?'

" 'Interested!' I shouted. My fingers shook so much that I could hardly dial Michael at the office. I met Michael at the agency and—well, here he is: Tommy." She held their son up for all to see.

Shelley and Michael had been through so much, and when they finally decided she would have a hysterectomy, I was fearful that both of them might give up on being parents. Staying with the RESOLVE group was the best thing they did for their marriage and for their happiness.

"I really don't know what to say." I took a sip of water to clear my throat. "You all worked so hard." I glanced around the table at their beaming faces. "We went through some tough times together. And now you seem so happy."

"In some ways I feel more fortunate than other couples," Margaret said. "But don't get me wrong; I wouldn't want to wish in vitro treatments on anyone."

"Right!" Kathy laughed.

As I listened to Margaret speak, I recalled how disappointed they were after her tubal surgery failed. She told me that before they decided what to do next, they repeated taking my "Why Is It So Important for You to Have a Baby?" test. Because of her age, and their determination to have their own baby, they decided to get into an in vitro program right away. Margaret never let any grass grow under her feet.

"But I learned something from all of this," Margaret said. "I discovered how strong our marriage really is, and I found out how really precious a baby can be."

Debbie raised her glass for a toast. "I'll second that."

"Just a minute, I'm not through," Margaret interrupted. "And I learned the importance of having a good doctor at your side." She turned toward me. "One who always seemed to have time to answer our questions, who helped us take control of our treatment, and who kept our spirits up."

"To Dr. Perloe." They raised their glasses in unison.

"To some very special people"—I glanced at the babies seated around the table—"and to some very special miracle babies."

It is to couples like these that I dedicate my book.

Appendixes

Appendix A:
A Letter to Family
and Friends

Dear Friend:

I realize that sometimes it's difficult for you to know what to say to a couple who has a fertility problem. Sometimes it seems like no matter what you do, it's the wrong thing. I'd like to give you a few suggestions that may help you be the friend I know you want to be:

1. *Be ready to listen.* Infertile couples have a lot on their minds and need someone to talk to. Sometimes a good ear helps people get things off their chests. A good listener can help people express their anxiety, anger, and guilt; or help people work out solutions to problems. Without offering any suggestions your attentiveness and interest may provide the comfort and reassurance these couples need most.

2. *Don't offer advice unless you are really well informed.* Infertile couples read everything they can get their hands on. Sometimes it seems as though they know more about fertility treatment than their own doctors. So talking off the cuff about something you don't really know about will only make them angry and defensive.

3. *Be sensitive and don't joke about infertility;* attempts at levity will only anger them. Joking about infertility is as inappropriate as joking about death at a funeral. Remember, infertile couples are hypersensitive about many things. Try to put yourself in their shoes whenever you insist they come to a baby shower, when you brag about your children's achievements, or when you tell them about your friend's daughter who got pregnant at fourteen.

4. *Be patient.* This couple may experience mood swings with every treatment or monthly cycle. One week they may be high because a new treatment promises hope; the next week they may be in mourning for the child they lost (didn't make) this month. They may be riding an exhausting emotional roller coaster which makes their actions and moods unpredictable. Try to under-

stand and flow with their changes. And remember that when they want to be alone, they are not rejecting you. Don't get your feelings hurt by the preoccupation they have with their problems; keep in touch.

5. *Show that you understand their difficulty.* Say things like, "I know this is difficult for you," "I don't envy what you're going through," or, "If there is anything I can do to help, don't hesitate to ask." If you aren't sure about what they are experiencing, read some articles and books that discuss the emotional aspects of fertility problems.

6. *Be realistic and supportive of their decisions for or against fertility treatment.* Once they've reached a difficult decision, don't say, "Shouldn't you see another doctor?"; "Are you sure that you really want to adopt?"; or, "I'd never consider doing that!" These couples usually weigh each issue as though it were a life-or-death decision. Don't take their decisions lightly unless you have good reason to.

7. *Don't put down their doctor or choices for treatment.* Refrain from making comments like, "I never heard of a doctor doing that. Does he know what he's doing?" or, "You don't need surgery. What you need is a vacation." Unless, from your reading or experience, you are certain that their physician is not using accepted methods, keep quiet about these topics.

8. *Be truthful.* Don't, for example, try to hide a pregnancy in the family. The truth does not hurt, provided you are not brutally frank.

9. *Let them know when you don't know what to say.* The couple will appreciate your honesty and will probably suggest how you can help them in that particular situation, even if it means remaining quiet. Admitting *your* problem will help establish honest communication.

10. *Be an advocate for infertile couples.* Educate others and speak up for the couple's decisions. Promote your local RESOLVE chapter. If you do not have a support group in your community, help form one.

11. *Understand that individuals and couples respond to fertility problems differently.* Learn to recognize the normal emotional stages they are experiencing—denial, anger, depression, mourning, acceptance, and so forth. And realize that they may cycle through these stages with each new round of treatment and with each lost opportunity. Accept them when they are angry, accept them when they are depressed, and accept them when they feel guilty. Unless they remain in a single stage for a prolonged period of time, don't become overly concerned.

12. Above all, *be there when they need you and show them that you care.*

This is a stressful time for everyone. Don't underestimate how important you and your relationship are to this couple. Your understanding and support can make a significant difference during this difficult period.

With warmest regards,
Mark Perloe, M.D.

Appendix B:
Associations and Organizations Providing Services and Information for Fertility Problems

American Adoption Congress
P.O. Box 44040, L'Enfant Station
Washington, D.C. 20026

American College of Obstetricians and
  Gynecologists
600 Maryland Ave. S.W., Suite 300
Washington, D.C. 20024

American Fertility Society
2131 Magnolia Ave., Suite 201
Birmingham, AL 35256

Americans for International Aid and
  Adoption
877 South Adams, Suite 106
Birmingham, MI 48011

Barren Foundation
230 N. Michigan Ave.
Chicago, IL 60610

Center for Communications in
  Infertility
P.O. Box 516
Yorktown Heights, NY 10598

Children's Services International
3109 Maple Dr. N.E., Suite 408
Atlanta, GA 30305

Committee for Single Adoptive
  Parents
P.O. Box 15084
Chevy Chase, MD 20815

Edna Gladney Center
2300 Hemphill St.
Fort Worth, TX 76110

The Endometriosis Association
P.O. Box 92187
Milwaukee, WI 53202

Fertility Research Foundation
1430 Second Ave., Suite 103
New York, NY 10021

Hold International Children's Service,
  Inc.
P.O. Box 2880
Eugene, OR 97402

Surrogates:
Infertility Center of New York
149 E. 60 St., Suite 1204
New York, NY 10022

Laser Research Foundation
3439 Kabel Dr., Suite 14
New Orleans, LA 70114

March of Dimes Birth Defects
  Foundation
1275 Mamaroneck Ave.
White Plains, NY 10605

National Center for Surrogate
  Parenting
5530 Wisconsin Ave.
Chevy Chase, MD 20815

National Committee for Adoption
1346 Connecticut Ave. N.W.,
  Suite 326
Washington, D.C. 20036

National Research Foundation for
  Fertility
53 E. 96 St.
New York, NY 10128

North American Center on Adoption
67 Irving Pl.
New York, NY 10003

North American Council on
  Adoptable Children
810 8 St. N.W., Suite 703
Washington, D.C. 20006

Adoption:
OURS, Inc.
3307 Highway 100 North
Minneapolis, MN 55422

Pearl S. Buck Foundation
Green Hill Farms
Perkasie, PA 18944

Planned Parenthood Federation of
  America, Inc.
810 Seventh Ave.
New York, NY 10019

Project Orphans Abroad
4100 Franklin Blvd.
Cleveland, OH 44113

RESOLVE, Inc.
P.O. Box 474
Belmont, MA 02178

SAME Christian Resource
  Center, Inc.
P.O. Box 2344
Bismarck, ND 58502

Southern California Fertility Institute
12301 Wilshire Blvd., Suite 415
Los Angeles, CA 90025

Surrogate Family Services, Inc.
125 S. 7 St.
Louisville, KY 40202

Surrogate Mothering Ltd.
1528 Walnut St.
Philadelphia, PA 19102

Surrogate Parenting Associates, Inc.
Doctor's Office Building, Suite 222
250 Liberty St.
Louisville, KY 40202

Welcome House
P.O. Box 836
Doylestown, PA 18901

Glossary

Abortion, Habitual: A term referring to a condition where a woman has had three or more miscarriages.

Abortion, Incomplete: An abortion after which some tissue remains inside the uterus. A D&C must be performed to remove the tissue and prevent complications.

Abortion, Missed: An abortion where the fetus dies in the uterus but there is no bleeding or cramping. A D&C will be needed to remove the fetal remains and prevent complications.

Abortion, Spontaneous: A pregnancy loss during the first twenty weeks of gestation.

Abortion, Therapeutic: A procedure used to terminate a pregnancy before the fetus can survive on its own.

Abortion, Threatened: Spotting or bleeding that occurs early in the pregnancy. May progress to spontaneous abortion.

Acrosin Test: A test performed to measure sperm enzyme activity necessary for penetrating the outer layer of the egg (zona pellucida); a test used to assess sperm fertilization capacity.

ACTH: A hormone produced by the pituitary gland to stimulate the adrenal glands. Excessive levels may lead to fertility problems.

Adhesion: Scar tissue occurring in the abdominal cavity, fallopian tubes, or inside the uterus. Adhesions can interfere with transport of the egg and implantation of the embryo in the uterus.

Adrenal Androgens: Male hormones produced by the adrenal gland which, when found in excess, may lead to fertility problems in both men and women. Excess androgens in the woman may lead to the formation of male secondary sex characteristics and the suppression of LH and FSH production by the pituitary gland. Elevated levels of androgens may be found in women with polycystic ovaries, or with a tumor in the pituitary gland, adrenal gland, or ovary. May also be associated with excess prolactin levels.

AID (Artificial Insemination Donor): *See* Artificial Insemination Donor.

AIH (Artificial Insemination Homologous): *See* Artificial Insemination Homologous.

Alpha-fetoprotein Test (AFP): A blood test performed to evaluate the development of the fetus and to look for fetal abnormalities.

Amenorrhea: The cessation of the menstrual periods for six months or more at a time.

Amenorrhea, Primary: A term used to refer to a woman who has never menstruated.

Amenorrhea, Secondary: A term describing a woman who has menstruated at one time, but who has not had a period for six months or more.

Andrologist: A physician-scientist who performs laboratory evaluations of male fertility. May hold a Ph.D. degree instead of an M.D. Usually affiliated with a fertility treatment center working on in vitro fertilization.

Anorexia Nervosa: A life-threatening eating disorder; self-imposed starvation. Severe weight loss and malnutrition from this disorder cause anovulation.

Anovulation: The failure to ovulate; ovulatory failure.

Antibodies: Chemicals made by the body to fight or attack foreign substances entering the body. Normally they prevent infection; however, when they attack the sperm or fetus, they cause infertility. Sperm antibodies may be made by either the man or the woman.

Artificial Insemination (AI): The depositing of sperm in the vagina near the cervix or directly into the uterus, with the use of a syringe instead of by coitus. This technique is used to overcome sexual performance problems, to circumvent sperm-mucus interaction problems, to maximize the potential for poor semen, and for using donor sperm. *See also* Artificial Insemination Donor; Artificial Insemination Homologous.

Artificial Insemination Donor (AID): Artificial insemination with donor sperm. A fresh donor semen specimen or a thawed frozen specimen is injected next to the woman's cervix.

Artificial Insemination Homologous (AIH): Artificial insemination with the husband's sperm. The sperm may be washed and injected directly into the wife's uterus (IAIH). Often used with poor semen or to overcome sperm-mucus problems.

Artificial Spermatocoele: An artificial, surgically created pouch used to collect sperm from men with irreversible tubal blockage.

Asherman's Syndrome: A condition where the uterine walls adhere to one another. Usually caused by uterine inflammation.

Asthenospermia: Low sperm motility.

Azospermia: Semen containing no sperm, either because the testicles cannot make sperm or because of blockage in the reproductive tract.

BBT Chart: A graph of the basal body temperature throughout the menstrual cycle. Shows the early morning temperature, the days the couple have sex, the days of menstrual flow, the time of mittleschmerz (if noted), the days that medication or fertility procedures are performed, and the days the woman may be ill, not feeling well, or running a fever. Used to document the likelihood that intercourse or insemination took place at the correct time.

Basal Body Temperature: The body temperature at complete rest. The woman's BBT is approximately one-half degree warmer during the latter half of her menstrual cycle than during the first half. This is due to the effects of progesterone secreted by the corpus luteum, which forms after ovulation.

Basal Body Temperature, Biphasic: A basal body temperature pattern consistent with ovulation and the formation of the corpus luteum, which secretes progesterone. This hormone will elevate the basal body temperature about one-half degree during the latter half of the menstrual cycle.

Basal Body Temperature, Monophasic: An anovulatory basal body temperature pattern where the temperature remains relatively constant throughout the cycle.

Beta hCG Test: A blood test used to detect very early pregnancies and to evaluate embryonic development.

Bicornuate Uterus: A congenital malformation of the uterus where the upper portion (horn) is duplicated.

Bromocriptine (Parlodel): An oral medication used to reduce prolactin. May also reduce the size of a pituitary tumor when present.

Bulimia: An eating disorder characterized by voracious eating followed by forced vomiting. The resulting weight loss and malnutrition may cause anovulation.

Buserelin: An experimental medication used for controlling endometriosis; long-acting GnRH available in a nasal spray and used to create the pseudomenopause desirable for reducing the size and number of endometriotic lesions.

Candidiasis (Yeast): An infection that may be uncomfortable and itchy and may impair fertility.

Capacitation: A process that sperm undergo as they travel through the woman's reproductive tract. Capacitation enables the sperm to penetrate the egg.

Cauterize: To burn tissue with electrical current (electrocautery) or with a laser. Used in surgical procedures to remove unwanted tissue such as adhesions and endometrial implants. Also used to control bleeding.

Cervical Mucus: A viscous fluid plugging the opening of the cervix. Most of the time this thick mucus plug prevents sperm and bacteria from entering the womb. However, at midcycle, under the influence of estrogen, the mucus becomes thin, watery, and stringy to allow sperm to pass into the womb. *See also* Cervix.

Cervical Smear: A sample of the cervical mucus examined microscopically to assess the presence of estrogen (ferning) and white blood cells, indicating possible infection.

Cervical Stenosis: A blockage of the cervical canal from a congenital defect or from complications of surgical procedures. *See also* Cervix.

Cervix: The opening between the uterus and the vagina. The cervical mucus plugs the cervical canal and normally prevents foreign materials from entering the reproductive tract. The cervix remains closed during pregnancy and dilates during labor and delivery to allow the baby to be born. *See also* Cervical Mucus; Cervix, Incompetent.

Cervix, Incompetent: A weakened cervix, which may allow the fetus to slip out of the uterus prematurely. This occurs during the second or third trimester.

Chocolate Cyst: A cyst in the ovary that is filled with old blood; endometrioma. Occurring when endometriosis invades an ovary, it causes the ovary to swell.

Chromosome: The structures in the cell that carry the genetic material (genes); the genetic messengers of inheritance. The human has forty-six chromosomes, twenty-three coming from the egg and twenty-three coming from the sperm.

Cilia: Tiny hairlike projections lining the inside surface of the fallopian tubes. The waving action of these "hairs" sweeps the egg toward the uterus.

Clitoris: The small erectile sex organ of the female which contains large numbers of sensory nerves; the female counterpart of the penis.

Clomid: *See* Clomiphene Citrate.

Clomiphene Citrate (Serophene, Clomid): A medication used to enhance pulsatile GnRH secretion from the hypothalamus. By "beating the drum" harder, the hypothalamus stimulates the pituitary to secrete FSH and LH, which stimulate the gonads. Serophene works well to induce ovulation in the woman who can produce estrogen. Marginal improvement in sperm production has been noted in some men taking the drug.

Coitus: Intercourse; the sexual union between a man and a woman.

Conception: *See* Fertilization.

Conceptus: The early products of conception; the embryo and placenta.

Condom Therapy: Therapy prescribed to reduce the number of sperm antibodies in the woman by using a condom during intercourse for six months or more and by the woman refraining from all skin contact with the husband's sperm. The woman's antibody level may fall to levels that will not adversely affect the sperm.

Cone Biopsy: A surgical procedure used to remove precancerous cells from the cervix. The procedure may damage the cervix and thus disrupt normal mucus production or cause an incompetent cervix, which may open prematurely during pregnancy.

Congenital Adrenal Hyperplasia: A congenital condition characterized by elevated androgens which suppress the pituitary gland and interfere with spermatogenesis or ovulation. Women may have ambiguous genitalia from the excess production of male hormone.

Contraception: The use of a method, medication, or device that will prevent pregnancy, such as condom, oral contraceptives, diaphragms, natural family planning, IUDs, spermicides, and sponges.

Contraceptive, Oral: A medication that prevents ovulation and pregnancy. Up to 3 percent of women taking the Pill will become anovulatory when they stop taking it. The regulatory effects of the Pill can also disguise symptoms of fertility problems— for example, an irregular cycle or endometriosis. May be used to control the symptoms and development of endometriosis.

Corpus Luteum: The yellow-pigmented glandular structure that forms from the ovarian follicle following ovulation. The gland produces progesterone, which is responsible for preparing and supporting the uterine lining for implantation. Progesterone also causes the half-degree basal temperature elevation noted at midcycle during an ovulatory cycle. If the corpus luteum functions poorly, the uterine lining may not support a pregnancy. If the egg is fertilized, a corpus luteum of pregnancy forms to maintain the endometrial bed and support the implanted embryo.

Cumulus Oophorus: The protective layer of cells surrounding the egg.

Cushing's Syndrome: A condition characterized by an overproduction of adrenal gland secretions. The person will suffer from high blood pressure and water retention as well as a number of other symptoms. A concurrent elevation of adrenal androgens will suppress pituitary output of LH and FSH and result in low sperm production or ovulatory failure. A woman may also develop male secondary sex characteristics, including abnormal hair growth. Cushing's Disease is another condition in which these same symptoms occur, but as the result of a pituitary tumor.

D&C (Dilation and Curettage): A procedure used to dilate the cervical canal and scrape out the lining and contents of the uterus. The procedure can be used to diagnose or treat the cause of abnormal bleeding and to terminate an unwanted pregnancy.

Danazol: A medication used to treat endometriosis. Suppresses LH and FSH production by the pituitary and causes a state of amenorrhea during which the endometrial implants waste away.

Delayed Ejaculation: A condition in which the man fakes orgasm and does not actually ejaculate when having sex.

Delayed Puberty: A condition in which the youngster fails to complete puberty and develop secondary sex characteristics by sixteen years of age. Puberty may be stimulated with hormonal replacement therapy. Some will outgrow the condition without treatment.

DES (Diethylstilbestrol): A medication prescribed in the 1950s and 1960s to women to prevent miscarriage. Male and female fetuses exposed in utero to this drug developed numerous deformities including blockage of the vas deferens, uterine abnormalities, cervical deformities, miscarriages, and unexplained infertility. DES is no longer prescribed for this indication.

DHEAS: *See* Adrenal Androgens.

Doxycycline: A tetracycline derivative; an antibiotic that inhibits many of the microorganisms infecting the reproductive tract. Often used for treating ureaplasma infections.

Dysmenorrhea: Painful menstruation. This may be a sign of endometriosis.

Dyspareunia: Painful coitus for either the man or the woman.

Ectopic Pregnancy: A pregnancy implanting outside of the uterus—for example, attached to the inside of the fallopian tube or to the ovary.

Egg Retrieval: A procedure used to obtain eggs from ovarian follicles for use in in vitro fertilization. The procedure may be performed during laparoscopy or by using a long needle and ultrasound to locate the follicle in the ovary.

Egg Transfer: *See* Embryo Transfer.

Ejaculate: The semen and sperm expelled during ejaculation.

Ejaculation: The physiological process by which the semen is propelled from the testicles, through the reproductive tract, and out the opening of the penis.

Embryo: The early products of conception; the undifferentiated beginnings of a baby; the conceptus.

Embryo Transfer: A procedure used to place a living embryo into a woman's uterus. The embryo may be a product of in vitro fertilization with her egg and her husband's sperm; or it may be an embryo washed from the womb of a surrogate.

Empty Sella Syndrome: A condition that occurs when spinal fluid leaks into the bony chamber (fossa) housing the pituitary gland. The fluid pressure compresses the pituitary gland and may adversely affect its ability to secrete LH and FSH and may elevate prolactin levels.

Endometrial Biopsy: A procedure during which a sample of the uterine lining is collected for microscopic analysis. The biopsy results will confirm ovulation and the proper preparation of the endometrium by estrogen and progesterone stimulation.

Endometriosis: A condition where endometrial tissue is located outside the womb. The tissue may attach itself to the reproductive organs or to other organs in the abdominal cavity. Each month the endometrial tissue "bleeds" with the onset of menses. The resultant irritation causes adhesions in the abdominal cavity and in the fallopian tubes. Endometriosis may also interfere with ovulation and with the implantation of the embryo.

Endometrium: The lining of the uterus which grows and sheds in response to estrogen and progesterone stimulation; the bed of tissue designed to nourish the implanted embryo.

Endorphins: Natural narcotics manufactured in the brain to reduce sensitivity to pain and stress. May contribute to stress-related fertility problems.

Epididymis: A coiled, tubular organ attached to and lying on the testicle. Within this organ the developing sperm complete their maturation and develop their powerful swimming capabilities. The matured sperm leave the epididymis through the vas deferens.

Erection: The process during which the erectile tissue of the penis becomes engorged with blood, causing the penis to swell and become rigid.

Estrogen: The female hormone produced in the ovary. Responsible for formation of the female secondary sex characteristics such as large breasts; supports the growth of the follicle and the development of the uterine lining. At midcycle the peak estrogen level triggers the release of the LH spike from the pituitary gland. The LH spike is necessary for the release of the ovum from the follicle. Fat cells in both obese men and women can also manufacture estrogen from androgens and interfere with fertility.

Expectant Therapy (Endometriosis): A wait-and-see approach used after laparoscopic surgery for mild endometriosis.

Fallopian Tubes: The two tubes leading from the uterus to the ovary through which the egg travels toward the uterus. Fertilization takes place within the tube.

Female Kallman's Syndrome: A condition characterized by infantile sexual development and an inability to smell. Since the pituitary cannot produce LH and FSH, the woman must take hormone supplements to achieve puberty, to maintain secondary sex characteristics, and to achieve fertility.

Ferning: A pattern characteristic of dried cervical mucus viewed on a slide. When the fern pattern appears, the mucus has been thinned and prepared by estrogen for the passage of sperm. If it does not fern, the mucus will be hostile to the passage of the sperm.

Fertile Eunuch: A rare disorder characterized by an LH deficiency leading to low testosterone levels and poor sperm production. Male secondary sex characteristics will be incomplete and sex drive will be low.

Fertility Specialist: A physician specializing in the practice of fertility. The American Board of Obstetrics and Gynecology certifies a subspecialty for OB-GYNs who receive extra training in endocrinology (the study of hormones) and infertility.

Fertility Treatment: Any method or procedure used to enhance fertility or increase the likelihood of pregnancy, such as ovulation induction treatment, varicocoele repair, and microsurgery to repair damaged fallopian tubes. The goal of fertility treatment is to help couples have a child.

Fertility Workup: The initial medical examinations and tests performed to diagnose or narrow down the cause of fertility problems.

Fertilization: The combining of the genetic material carried by sperm and egg to create an embryo. Normally occurs inside the fallopian tube (in vivo) but may also occur in a petri dish (in vitro). *See also* In Vitro Fertilization.

Fetus: A term used to refer to a baby during the period of gestation between eight weeks and term.

Fibroid (Leiomyomata): A benign muscle tumor of the uterus which may affect fertility.

Fimbria: The opening of the fallopian tube near the ovary. When stimulated by the follicular fluid released during ovulation, the fingerlike ends grasp the ovary and coax the egg into the tube.

Fimbrioplasty: *See* Salpingostomy/Fimbrioplasty.

Fitzhugh-Curtis Syndrome: Adhesions that attach the liver to the inside of the abdominal wall. A condition that can be caused by pelvic inflammatory disease (PID).

Follicle: A fluid-filled capsule that surrounds the ovum while it is developing in the ovary.

Follicular Fluid: The fluid inside the follicle that cushions and nourishes the ovum. When released during ovulation, the fluid stimulates the fimbria to grasp the ovary and coax the egg into the fallopian tube.

Follicular Phase: The first half of the menstrual cycle during which the follicle develops and the ovum matures.

FSH (Follicle-Stimulating Hormone): A pituitary hormone that stimulates spermatogenesis and follicular development. In the man FSH stimulates the Sertoli cells in the testicles and supports sperm production. In the woman FSH stimulates the growth of the ovarian follicle. Elevated FSH levels are indicative of gonadal failure in both men and woman.

Galactorrhea: A clear or milky discharge from the breasts associated with elevated prolactin.

Gamete Intrafallopian Transfer (GIFT): A new technique that may be used in lieu of in vitro fertilization for women with patent tubes. After egg retrieval the eggs are mixed with the husband's sperm and then injected through the fimbria into the woman's fallopian tubes for in vivo fertilization.

Gardnerella Infection: A vaginal infection that causes a burning sensation and a gray, malodorous discharge. May interfere with fertility.

General Practitioner: A family physician who can assess your general health and investigate the potential effects of medical history, environment, and medications on your fertility.

Genitals: The external sex organs, as the labia and clitoris in the woman and the penis and testicles in the man. Also called genitalia.

Germ Cell: In the male the testicular cell that divides to produce the immature sperm cells; in the woman the ovarian cell that divides to form the egg (ovum). The male germ cell remains intact throughout the man's reproductive life; the woman uses up her germ cells at the rate of about one thousand per menstrual cycle, although usually only one egg matures each cycle.

Germ Cell Aplasia (Sertoli Cell Only); An inherited condition in which the testicles have no germ cells. Since men with this condition have normal Leydig cells, they will develop secondary sex characteristics. May also be caused by large and/or prolonged exposure to toxins or radiation.

GnRH (Gonadotropic-Releasing Hormone): A substance secreted by the hypothalamus every ninety minutes or so. This hormone enables the pituitary to secrete LH and FSH, which stimulate the gonads. *See also* FSH; LH.

Gonad: The gland that makes reproductive cells and "sex" hormones, as the testicles, which make sperm and testosterone, and the ovaries, which make eggs (ova) and estrogen.

Gonorrhea: An infection that is usually asymptomatic, but that may cause a bad-smelling yellowish vaginal discharge and red and swollen vaginal walls. If it reaches the fallopian tubes, the woman will suffer pain, develop a high fever, and possibly develop tubal blockage. The responsible organism may also impair sperm and prevent pregnancy. In the man gonorrhea seldom leads to damage, but it may cause a painful infection.

Habitual Abortion: *See* Abortion, Habitual.

hCG (Human Chorionic Gonadotropin): A medication used to release the egg from the follicle. May also be used to stimulate sexual development when the pituitary gland fails. Normally hCG is secreted by the placenta to preserve pregnancy.

Hamster Penetration Test: A test performed to predict if sperm are capable of fertilizing an egg.

Hepatitis: Liver disease. The liver filters impurities from the blood, including "old" hormones. When this system breaks down, elevated estrogen levels may interfere with ovulation.

Hirsutism: The overabundance of body hair, such as a mustache or pubic hair growing upward toward the navel, found in women with excess androgens.

hMG: *See* Pergonal.

Hyperprolactinemia: A condition in which the pituitary gland secretes too much prolactin. Prolactin can suppress LH and FSH production, reduce sex drive in the man, and directly suppress ovarian function in the woman.

Hyperstimulation: A potentially life-threatening side effect of Pergonal ovulation induction treatment. Arises when too many follicles develop and hCG is given to release the eggs. May be prevented by withholding the hCG injection when ultrasound monitoring indicates that too many follicles have matured.

Hypertension: High blood pressure.

Hyperthyroidism: Overproduction of thyroid hormone by the thyroid gland. The resulting increased metabolism "burns up" estrogen too rapidly and interferes with ovulation.

Hypoestrogenic: Having lower than normal levels of estrogen.

Hypogonadotropic Hypopituitarism: A spectrum of diseases resulting in low pituitary gland output of LH and FSH. Men with this disorder have low sperm counts and may lose their virility; women do not ovulate and may lose their secondary sex characteristics.

Hypospermatogenesis: Low sperm production.

Hypothalamus: A part of the brain, the hormonal regulation center, located adjacent to and above the pituitary gland. In both the man and the woman this tissue secretes GnRH every ninety minutes or so. The pulsatile GnRH enables the pituitary gland to secrete LH and FSH, which stimulate the gonads. *See also* FSH; LH; Ovary; Pituitary Gland; Testicle.

Hypothyroidism: A condition in which the thyroid gland produces an insufficient amount of thyroid hormone. The resulting lowered metabolism interferes with the normal breakdown of "old" hormones and causes lethargy. Men will suffer from a lower sex drive and elevated prolactin (*see* Hyperprolactinemia), and women will suffer from elevated prolactin and estrogen, both of which will interfere with fertility.

Hysterectomy: The surgical removal of the uterus. May also include the removal of other reproductive structures, such as the fallopian tubes and ovaries.

Hysterosalpingogram (HSG, Hysterogram); An X ray of the inside of the uterus and tubes. To highlight the hollow interior structure, a dye is injected through the cervix. If the dye pours through the fallopian tubes into the abdomen, the tubes are open (patent).

Hysteroscope: A small telescope used to look inside the cervical canal and uterus. The procedure is called a hysteroscopy. May be used in conjunction with surgical instruments to remove intrauterine adhesions and fibroids.

Hysteroscopy: A procedure performed to diagnose fertility problems caused by abnormalities inside the uterine cavity. A hysteroscope is slipped through the cervix to view the inside of the uterus directly.

IAIH (Intrauterine Artificial Insemination Homologous): Artificial insemination where the husband's sperm is injected directly into the uterus to avoid cervical mucus problems or to maximize the potential for poor semen. *See also* Artificial Insemination.

Immature Sperm (Germinal Cell): A sperm that has not matured and gained the ability to swim. In the presence of illness or infection such sperm may appear in the semen in large numbers.

Imperforate Hymen: A condition where the membrane (hymen) covering the vagina fails to open and allow menstrual flow.

Implantation (Embryo): The embedding of the embryo into tissue so it can establish contact with the mother's blood supply for nourishment. Implantation usually occurs in the lining of the uterus; however, in an ectopic pregnancy it may occur elsewhere in the body.

Impotence: The inability of the man to have an erection and to ejaculate.

In Vitro Fertilization: A technique for retrieving the woman's eggs and mixing them with her husband's sperm in a petri dish. Once the eggs are fertilized, the embryos are transferred to her womb for implantation. Frequently used to resolve tubal problems or problems with poor semen.

Incompetent Cervix: *See* Cervix, Incompetent.

Infertility: The inability to conceive after a year of unprotected intercourse or the inability to carry a pregnancy to term.

Inhibin: A male feedback hormone made in the testicles to regulate FSH production by the pituitary gland.

Inhibin-F (Folliculostatin): A female feedback hormone made in the ovary to regulate FSH production by the pituitary gland.

IUD (Intrauterine Device): A device placed into the uterus to prevent pregnancy. The IUD has been associated with an increased incidence of infection, which may damage the fallopian tubes, and is therefore not recommended for women with multiple sexual partners.

Kallman's Syndrome: A congenital hypothalamic dysfunction which has multiple symptoms including the failure to complete puberty.

Karyotyping: A test performed to analyze chromosomes for the presence of genetic defects.

Klinefelter's Syndrome: A genetic abnormality characterized by having one Y (male) and two X (female) chromosomes. May cause a fertility problem.

Laparoscope: A small telescope that can be inserted into a hole in the abdominal wall for viewing the internal organs; the instrument used to perform a laparoscopy. Used to diagnose and treat a number of fertility problems including endometriosis, abdominal adhesions, and polycystic ovaries. Also used in egg retrieval for in vitro fertilization.

Laparoscopy: A surgical procedure done under general anesthesia. A small telescope is slipped through a tiny incision in the belly button. Through the laparoscope the surgeon can view the abdominal organs to diagnose fertility problems. Some surgical procedures such as the removal of filmy adhesions may be done during the procedure.

Laparotomy: Major abdominal surgery where reproductive organ abnormalities can be corrected and fertility restored, such as tubal repairs and the removal of adhesions.

Lavage: *See* Uterine Lavage.

Leiomyomata: *See* Fibroid.

Leydig Cell: The testicular cell that produces the male hormone testosterone. The Leydig cell is stimulated by LH from the pituitary gland.

LH (Luteinizing Hormone): A pituitary hormone that stimulates the gonads. In the man LH is necessary for spermatogenesis (Sertoli cell function) and for the production of testosterone (Leydig cell function). In the woman LH is necessary for the production of estrogen. When estrogen reaches a critical peak, the pituitary releases a surge of LH (the LH spike), which releases the egg from the follicle.

LH Spike (Surge): A sudden release of LH from the pituitary gland at midcycle. Triggered when estrogen reaches a critical peak, the LH spike releases the egg from the follicle. *See also* LH.

Lumen: The hollow chamber inside a tube, such as the channel inside the fallopian tube or vas deferens.

Luteal Phase: The latter half of the menstrual cycle which follows ovulation. During the luteal phase the corpus luteum forms and produces progesterone.

Luteal Phase Defect (LPD): A condition that occurs when the uterine lining does not develop adequately because of inadequate progesterone stimulation; or because of the inability of the uterine lining to respond to progesterone stimulation. LPD may prevent embryonic implantation or cause an early abortion.

Luteinized Unruptured Follicles: A condition in which the follicle develops and changes into the corpus luteum without releasing the egg.

Masturbation: A technique used to collect semen for analysis and for artificial insemination; manual stimulation of the penis leading to ejaculation.

Maturation Arrest: A testicular condition in which at one stage of sperm production all sperm development halts throughout all testicular tubules. May result in oligospermia or azospermia.

Meiosis: The cell division, peculiar to reproductive cells, which allows genetic material to divide in half. Each new cell will contain twenty-three chromosomes. The spermatids (immature sperm) and ova (eggs) each contain twenty-three chromosomes, so when they combine (fertilize), the baby will have a normal complement of forty-six.

Menorrhagia: Heavy or prolonged menstrual flow.

Menstruation: The cyclical shedding of the uterine lining in response to stimulation from estrogen and progesterone.

Metrorrhagia: Menstrual spotting during the middle of the cycle.

Miscarriage: Spontaneous loss of an embryo or fetus from the womb.

Mitosis: The division of a cell into two identical cells in which all forty-six human chromosomes are duplicated; the first division of the germ cell.

Mittleschmerz: The discomfort felt on one side of the lower abdomen at the time of ovulation.

Morphology, Sperm: The form or shape of the sperm cell. An evaluation performed during the semen analysis to determine the number of "normal" sperm in the sample.

Motility, Sperm: The ability of the sperm to swim in a straight line. An evaluation performed during the semen analysis. The semen analysis factor most highly correlated with fertility.

Mycoplasma: *See* Ureaplasma.

Myomectomy: Surgery performed to remove fibroid tumors.

Newborn Death: The death of a baby within the first month after birth.

Obstetrician-Gynecologist: A specialist in the study and treatment of women's diseases, especially of the genitourinary and rectal tracts. In addition, these physicians are concerned with the treatment of women during pregnancy and childbirth.

Oligospermia: A sperm count below 20 million; a low sperm count; a sperm count low enough to cause a fertility problem.

Orgasm: The psychological and physical thrill that accompanies sexual climax. For the man orgasm causes ejaculation.

Ovarian Cyst: A fluid-filled sac inside the ovary. An ovarian cyst may be found in conjunction with ovulation disorders, tumors of the ovary, and endometriosis. *See also* Chocolate Cyst.

Ovarian Failure: The failure of the ovary to respond to FSH stimulation from the pituitary because of damage to or malformation of the ovary. Diagnosed by elevated FSH in the blood.

Ovulation: The release of the egg (ovum) from the ovarian follicle.

Ovulation Induction: Medical treatment performed to initiate ovulation. *See also* Clomiphene Citrate; Pergonal.

Ovulatory Failure (Anovulation): The failure to ovulate.

Ovum: The egg; the reproductive cell from the ovary; the female gamete; the sex cell that contains the woman's genetic information.

Panhypopituitarism: Complete pituitary gland failure.

Parlodel: *See* Bromocriptine.

Patent: The condition of being open, as with tubes that form part of the reproductive organs.

Penile Implant: A device surgically inserted into the penis to provide rigidity for intercourse. Used to treat impotence.

Penis: The male organ that becomes enlarged and erect for the purpose of depositing semen in the woman's vagina.

Pergonal (hMG, Human Menopausal Gonadotropin): A medication used to replace the pituitary hormones, LH and FSH. May be used to induce ovulation in women who do not respond to clomiphene citrate. Most frequently used with women who do not normally produce estrogen because of a pituitary gland or hypothalamic malfunction. May also be used with men to stimulate sperm production.

PID (Pelvic Inflammatory Disease): An infection of the pelvic organs that causes severe illness, high fever, and extreme pain. PID may lead to tubal blockage and pelvic adhesions.

Pituitary Gland: The master gland; the gland that is stimulated by the hypothalamus and controls all hormonal functions. Located at the base of the brain just below the hypothalamus, this gland controls many major hormonal factories throughout the body including the gonads, the adrenal glands, and the thyroid gland.

Placenta: The embryonic tissue that invades the uterine wall and provides a mechanism for exchanging the baby's waste products for the mother's nutrients and oxygen. The baby is connected to the placenta by the umbilical cord.

Polar Body: The discarded genetic material resulting from female germ cell division. *See also* Meiosis.

Polycystic Ovaries: A condition seen with anovulation where many small cysts develop in the ovary. The degenerating follicles (cysts) continue to secrete androgen and thus interfere with subsequent ovulation.

Postcoital Test: A microscopic examination of the cervical mucus to determine compatibility between the woman's mucus and the man's semen; a test used to detect sperm-mucus interaction problems, the presence of sperm antibodies, and the quality of the cervical mucus.

Posttesticular System: The ducts that store and deliver the sperm to the opening of the penis; also includes the glands that produce seminal fluids.

Pregnancy Test: A test used to determine if a woman is pregnant. A new home pregnancy test such as the Tambrands First Response™ Pregnancy Test can detect a pregnancy on the first day that the menstrual period fails to begin.

Premature Ejaculation: A condition in which the man becomes so sexually excited that most of the time he ejaculates prior to penetrating the woman's vagina.

Premature Ovarian Failure: A condition where the ovary runs out of follicles before the normal age associated with menopause.

Pretesticular System: The male hormonal system responsible for stimulating sperm production and the development of male secondary sex characteristics.

Progesterone: A hormone secreted by the corpus luteum during the latter half of the menstrual cycle. The hormone helps prepare the uterine lining for implantation and also helps maintain a pregnancy.

Progesterone Withdrawal: A diagnostic procedure used to analyze menstrual irregularity and amenorrhea; uterine "bleeding" that occurs within two weeks after taking progesterone; a procedure used to demonstrate the presence or absence of estrogen and to demonstrate the ability of the uterus and reproductive tract to "bleed." Prior to ovulation induction therapy, progesterone withdrawal may be used to induce a menstrual period.

Prostaglandin: A hormone secreted by the uterine lining. It is hypothesized that prostaglandins secreted by active, young endometrial implants may interfere with the reproductive organs by causing muscular contractions or spasms.

Prostate Gland: A gland in the male reproductive system that produces a portion of the semen including a chemical that liquefies the coagulated semen twenty minutes to one hour after entering the vagina.

Puberty: The time of life when the body begins making adult levels of sex hormones (estrogen or testosterone) and the youngster takes on adult body characteristics: developing breasts, growing a beard, pubic hair, and auxiliary hair; attaining sexual maturity.

Refractory Period: A period of time after orgasm during which a man or woman cannot have another; a recovery period.

Resistant Ovary: An ovary that cannot respond to the follicle-stimulating message sent by FSH. Primitive germ cells will be present in the ovary; however, they will not respond to FSH stimulation.

Retrograde Ejaculation: A male fertility problem that allows the sperm to travel into the bladder instead of out the opening of the penis due to a failure in the sphincter muscle at the base of the bladder.

Rubin's Test: A procedure used in the past to determine if the fallopian tubes were open. Pressurized carbon dioxide was forced through the cervix. If the tubes were open, the gas would pass through the fallopian tubes and into the abdominal cavity. The test is no longer used, since the hysterosalpingogram provides so much more information.

Salpingectomy: Surgical removal of the fallopian tube.

Salpingolysis: Surgery performed to remove adhesions that restrict the movement and function of reproductive organs.

Salpingostomy/Fimbrioplasty: Surgical repair made to the fallopian tubes; a procedure used to open the fimbria.

Scrotum: The bag of skin and thin muscle surrounding the man's testicles.

Secondary Sex Characteristics: The physical qualities that distinguish man and woman, such as beard, large breasts, and deep voice. Formed under the stimulation of the sex hormones (testosterone or estrogen), these characteristics also identify those people who have gone through puberty (sexual maturity).

Semen: The fluid portion of the ejaculate consisting of secretions from the seminal vesicles, prostate gland, and several other glands in the male reproductive tract. The semen provides nourishment and protection for the sperm and a medium in which the sperm can travel to the woman's vagina. Semen may also refer to the entire ejaculate, including the sperm.

Semen Analysis: A laboratory test used to assess semen quality: sperm quantity, concentration, morphology (form), and motility. In addition, it measures semen (fluid) volume and whether or not white blood cells are present, indicating an infection.

Semen Viscosity: The liquid flow or consistency of the semen.

Seminal Vesicles: Glands in the male reproductive system which produce much of the semen volume, including fructose (sugar) for nourishing the sperm and a chemical that causes the semen to coagulate on entering the vagina.

Seminiferous Tubes: The testicular tubules in which the sperm mature and move toward the epididymis.

Septate Uterus: A uterus divided into right and left halves by a wall of tissue (septum). Women with a septate uterus have an increased chance of early pregnancy loss.

Serophene: *See* Clomiphene Citrate.

Sertoli (Nurse) Cell: A testicular cell responsible for nurturing the spermatids (immature sperm). Secretes inhibin, a feedback hormone, which regulates FSH production by the pituitary gland. When stimulated by FSH, the Sertoli cell initiates spermatogenesis.

Sheehan's Syndrome: A condition caused by profuse hemorrhage at the time of delivery. The severe blood loss shocks the pituitary gland, which dies and becomes nonfunctional.

Short Luteal Phase: A condition in which the corpus luteum deteriorates prematurely, causing the menstrual period to begin approximately ten days (instead of fourteen) after ovulation. Frequently found with women undergoing ovulation induction treatment.

Sperm: The microscopic cell that carries the male's genetic information to the female's egg; the male reproductive cell; the male gamete.

Sperm Agglutination: Sperm clumping caused by antibody reactions or by infection.

Sperm Antibodies: Antibodies that attack and maim sperm. May be formed by either the man against his own sperm or by the woman against her husband's sperm.

Sperm Bank: A registered tissue bank that collects, stores, tests, and sells sperm for artificial insemination.

Sperm Concentration: The number of sperm per volume of semen.

Sperm Maturation: A process during which the sperm grow and gain their ability to swim. Sperm take about ninety days to reach maturity.

Sperm Morphology: A semen analysis factor that indicates the number or percentage of sperm in the sample that appear to have been formed normally. Abnormal morphology includes sperm with kinked, doubled, or coiled tails.

Sperm-Mucus Cross Test: A test used to diagnose the presence of sperm antibodies. The man's sperm are placed in bovine mucus, donor sperm are placed in the woman's mucus, and the husband's sperm and wife's mucus are mixed together. Microscopic examination will reveal the source of the sperm antibodies.

Sperm-Mucus Interaction: *See* Postcoital Test.

Sperm Penetration: The ability of the sperm to penetrate the egg so it can deposit the genetic material during fertilization.

Spermatogenesis: Sperm production in the testicles.

Spinnbarkeit: The stretchability of cervical mucus; the stringy quality that occurs at midcycle under the influence of estrogen. *See also* Postcoital Test.

Split Ejaculate: A method used to concentrate the sperm for insemination; separating the semen into two portions: the first portion of the ejaculate, which is rich in sperm, and the second portion, which contains mostly seminal fluid.

Spontaneous Abortion: *See* Abortion, Spontaneous.

Stein-Leventhal Disease: Another name for polycystic ovaries.

Sterility: An irreversible condition that prevents conception.

Stillbirth: The death of a fetus between the twentieth week of gestation and birth.

Surrogate Mother: A woman who agrees to be inseminated with the husband's sperm and carry the baby to term. At birth she relinquishes the baby for adoption by the man and his wife.

Surrogate Womb: A woman who in effect "rents" her womb to a couple. The couple uses in vitro fertilization to "create" their own embryo, which is then transferred to the surrogate's womb for gestation.

Testicular Biopsy: A minor surgical procedure used to take a small sample of testicular tissue for microscopic examination; a test used to diagnose male fertility problems when no other means is available (this is because the biopsy procedure itself may cause testicular damage).

Testicular Enzyme Defect: A congenital enzyme defect that prevents the testes from responding to hormonal stimulation. Will result in oligospermia or azospermia.

Testicular Failure, Primary: A congenital, developmental, or genetic error resulting in a testicular malformation that prevents sperm production.

Testicular Failure, Secondary: Acquired testicular damage—for example, from drugs, prolonged exposure to toxic substances, or a varicocoele.

Testicular Feminization: An enzymatic defect that prevents a man from responding to the male hormone testosterone. The man will look like a woman, but karyotyping will reveal a normal XY male chromosome pattern, and testosterone levels will be in the normal male range.

Testicular Function: The ability of the testicles to produce sperm and testosterone.

Testicular Stress Pattern: A semen analysis result showing depressed sperm production, poor sperm motility, and poor sperm morphology. The pattern is consistent with secondary testicular failure or illness.

Testosterone: The male hormone responsible for the formation of secondary sex characteristics and for supporting the sex drive. Testosterone is also necessary for spermatogenesis.

Torsion: The twisting of the testis inside the scrotum. Besides causing extreme pain and swelling, the rotation twists off the blood supply and causes severe damage to the testicle. Torsion of the ovary may also occur in a woman suffering from hyperstimulation, a complication of ovulation induction treatment.

Trichomonas: An infection that may produce a greenish, bad-smelling vaginal discharge.

Tubocornual Anastomosis: Surgery performed to remove a blocked portion of the fallopian tube and to reconnect the tube to the uterus. Tubouterine implantation may also be performed to remove fallopian tube blockage near the uterus and reimplant the tube in the uterus.

Tubotubal Anastomosis: Surgery performed to remove a diseased portion of the fallopian tube and reconnect the two ends; sterilization reversal.

Turner's Syndrome: The most common genetic defect contributing to female fertility problems. The ovaries fail to form and appear as slender threads of atrophic ovarian tissue, referred to as streak ovaries. Karyotyping will reveal that this woman has only one female (X) chromosome instead of two.

Ultrasound: A test used instead of X rays to visualize the reproductive organs; for example, to monitor follicular development and to examine the tubes and uterus. The instrument works by bouncing sound waves off the organs. A picture displayed on a TV screen shows the internal organs.

Umbilical Cord: Two arteries and one vein encased in a gelatinous tube leading from the baby to the placenta. Used to exchange nutrients and oxygen from the mother for waste products from the baby.

Undescended Testicles (Cryptorchidism): The failure of the testicles to descend from the abdominal cavity into the scrotum by one year of age. If not repaired by age six, may result in permanent fertility loss.

Ureaplasma (Mycoplasma): An infection that may cause the formation of sperm antibodies and an inflammation of the uterine lining, either of which may interfere with implantation of the embryo.

Urethra: The tube that allows urine to pass between the bladder and the outside of the body. In the man this tube also carries semen from the area of the prostate to the outside.

Urologist: A physician specializing in the genitourinary tract.

Uterine Lavage: A technique used to wash an embryo from a donor's uterus in order to transfer it to an infertile woman.

Uterus: The hollow, muscular organ that houses and nourishes the fetus during pregnancy.

Vagina: The canal leading from the cervix to the outside of the woman's body; the birth passage.

Vaginitis: Yeast, gardnerella, or trichomonas infections of the vagina. Frequent vaginitis may indicate the presence of pelvic adhesions and tubal blockage from other infections, such as chlamydia. Vaginitis may interfere with sperm penetration of the cervical mucus, and the symptoms may even interfere with the ability and desire to have intercourse.

Varicocele: A dilation of the veins that carry blood out of the scrotum. The resulting swollen vessels surrounding the testicles create a pool of stagnant blood, which elevates the scrotal temperature. A major cause of male infertility.

Vas Deferens: One of the tubes through which the sperm move from the testicles (epididymis) toward the seminal vesicles and prostate gland. These tubes are severed during a vasectomy performed for birth control.

Vasectomy: The accidental or elective surgical separation of the vasa deferentia; a procedure used for birth control.

Venereal Disease: Any infection that can be sexually transmitted, such as chlamydia, gonorrhea, ureaplasma, and syphilis. Many of these diseases will interfere with fertility and some will cause severe illness. *See also* PID.

Virility: Masculinization; having male secondary sex characteristics; being able to perform sexually.

X Chromosome: The congenital, developmental, or genetic information in the cell that transmits the information necessary to make a female. All eggs contain one X chromosome, and half of all sperm carry an X chromosome. When two X chromosomes combine, the baby will be a girl. *See also* Y Chromosome.

Y Chromosome: The genetic material that transmits the information necessary to make a male. The Y chromosome can be found in one-half of the man's sperm cells. When an X and a Y chromosome combine, the baby will be a boy. *See also* X Chromosome.

Index